Skewed Studies

Skewed Studies

Exploring the Limits and Flaws of Health and Psychology Research

Sally Kuykendall

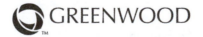 GREENWOOD

An Imprint of ABC-CLIO, LLC

Santa Barbara, California • Denver, Colorado

Library of Congress Cataloging in Publication Control Number: 2019057136

ISBN: 978-1-4408-6398-1 (print)
     978-1-4408-6399-8 (ebook)

24 23 22 21 20   1 2 3 4 5

This book is also available as an eBook.

Greenwood
An Imprint of ABC-CLIO, LLC

ABC-CLIO, LLC
147 Castilian Drive
Santa Barbara, California 93117
www.abc-clio.com

This book is printed on acid-free paper ∞

Manufactured in the United States of America

To my best friend and partner, Butch, and to all of the hard-working scientists who do what is right to advance humanity

Contents

Preface

As an undergraduate and graduate student, I was fortunate to have wonderful research mentors. My mentors taught me how to think creatively and strategically about pressing health issues, how to develop a realistic study proposal, and how to collaborate with others, collect data, and, most important, how to act with professionalism and integrity. My background in nursing helped. In nursing, honesty, integrity, and professionalism are essential to patient care. Nurses are required to report suspicions of professional misconduct. Failure to report could result in suspension of one's nursing license.

As part of the academic process, faculty members are required to review other faculty members. The first time I came across research misconduct was as a faculty member. I was shocked and disheartened. I distanced myself from the individual and the situation. The person eventually left the institution. The second time I discovered misconduct, I was less shocked. I quietly and confidentially advised the individual of what I had found. She lashed out, spreading nasty rumors. The third time I noticed research misconduct, I was warned to stay silent and advised that "everyone does it." "It" being research misconduct. Six weeks later, my annual review noted that I was a failure in service. The failure came out of the blue. I had never received any indication that my service was unsatisfactory. I started to realize that the response "everyone does it" may have been more a little more accurate than I wanted to believe. I was naive. My mentors had never schooled me on the fact that "everyone does it."

I am wiser now. What I experienced is nothing in comparison to the retaliation experienced by Walter DeNino, Tyler Shultz, Betty Dong, Nancy Olivieri, and Kenneth Sloane. *Skewed Studies: Exploring the Limits and Flaws of Health and Psychology Research* is in honor of students, would-be and actual whistle-blower and those who have suffered personal and professional attack because you thought science should be honest and that scientists should act with integrity. I believe that the best way to stop scientific misconduct is to speak out. Distancing ourselves, pushing the perpetrators along to the next institution, or subjecting students to dishonest practices will not eliminate the problem. Scientific misconduct harms science, scientists, and human progress. We must name the behaviors and identify the very real consequences of misconduct on patients, family members, and communities. If science is about a search for the truth, we cannot be afraid to speak the truth.

Acknowledgments

I am grateful to Dr. Alice Hausman of Temple University and Dr. G. Peter Matthews of the University of Plymouth (UK) for modeling high standards of scientific integrity. I am grateful to the courageous whistle-blowers who put their reputation and career on the line to halt misconduct. Without their voices and stories, this book could not exist. I am extremely grateful for the hundreds of articles and resources accessed through Drexel Library. The librarians were extremely patient with my many unusual requests. I am grateful to Dr. Jenny Spinner of Saint Joseph's University for sharing her expertise in journalism and to Professor David Kaye of Penn State University for sharing his adventures with flaky academic conference requests. As always, I am thankful to my wonderful husband, Butch, for listening, questioning, and supporting and my sons, Matthew, Mark, and Alex, and stepdaughters, Eva and Emily, for being there.

ONE

The Scientific Method

Science is an intellectual activity where the scientist systematically investigates facts, patterns, or laws related to nature or the world. The purpose of scientific investigation is to develop a body of knowledge in the particular area of interest. Developing this body of knowledge frees humanity from misconceptions or superstition and provides a foundation for advancement. Microbiology is a good example of the development of a body of knowledge that led to later advancements. Ancient civilizations believed that infectious diseases were punishment by supernatural beings for wrongdoing. Through repeated observation of patients and their surroundings, ancient Greek, Roman, and Chinese doctors developed miasma theory. Miasma theory proposed that bad air, not gods and goddesses, caused infectious diseases. In 1546, Italian physician Girolamo Fracastoro suggested that seedlike particles shared among people in close proximity were the source of infection. Antonie van Leeuwenhoek's invention of the microscope enabled scientists to create and confirm the germ theory of disease. Today, we have antibiotics, vaccinations, sterile surgical procedures, antiretroviral therapies, and infection control programs to prevent and limit infectious diseases. Thankfully, we have moved past the idea that polio, smallpox, cholera, and typhoid are caused by angry gods or goddesses. Thus, science is not just an intellectual activity. Science allows us to understand natural phenomenon, develop theories, and create tools that make lives better. Electricity, computers, cars, airplanes, sanitation, and medicine are all the result of scientific endeavors. Ultimately, science is a quest for the truth, truth about nature, truth about social behaviors, and truth about the universe.

Scientific endeavors can be very time-consuming. Three hundred years passed between Fracastoro's theory of seedlike particles and Dr. Ignaz Semmelweis's suggestion that doctors wash their hands before examining pregnant women, and even then, Semmelweis's suggestion was met with disdain and disbelief. The idea that highly respected gentlemen doctors carried germs was shocking and inconsistent with current theory of spontaneous generation. In order to advance a particular field, scientists must study previous work and ideas on the topic, deal with the frustration of failed experiments, check and recheck their findings, and confront mistrust or skepticism over study results. The *scientific method* is a systematic process used by scientists to minimize failure and avoid potential biases. The main steps of the scientific method are to: (a) identify the problem or phenomenon of interest; (b) assess existing knowledge of the phenomenon; (c) formulate a research question or research hypothesis; (d) plan an experiment; (e) collect data; (f) analyze results; and (g) draw logical conclusions. In practice, the method is complicated. Each part connects to the other parts to develop a cohesive line of inquiry. This methodical approach maximizes efficiency in building the body of knowledge. Without such a system, scientists would waste time and resources creating discoveries that already existed, gathering information that is already known, or proposing misleading theories. Later chapters explain each step of the scientific method in detail. This chapter presents an overview of the history of the scientific method and examples of exploitation of the scientific method.

DEVELOPMENT OF THE SCIENTIFIC METHOD IN HEALTH AND PSYCHOLOGY

The philosophy of science as a search for the truth is critical to understanding science and medical research. The scientific method traces back to the sixth century BCE in Anatolia, now the country of Turkey, and the innovative Milesian School. The school was founded by three philosophers, Thales of Miletus (c. 624–c. 546 BCE), Anaximander (c. 610–c. 546 BCE), and Anaximenes of Miletus (c. 585–c. 528 BCE). The premise of the school was controversial, even blasphemous for ancient times. Teachers encouraged students to set aside beliefs that gods and goddesses controlled weather, disease, and life events and instead to search for common patterns and characteristics in nature that may explain the phenomena. Wealthy patrons supported school staff and students in their studies with the expectation that students and teachers would investigate phenomena with honesty and integrity. Milesian theory spread, freeing Greek and Roman scientists to explore the world without fear. While Roman scientists sought practical knowledge, outcomes that would improve crops or advance the Roman Empire, Greek scientists sought knowledge for the sake of knowledge. Through these early investigations, ancient scholars created the foundations for astronomy, mathematics, biology, and agriculture. Other ancient philosophers, such as Socrates (c. 470–c. 399 BCE), Plato (c. 428–c. 348 BCE), and Aristotle (384–322 BCE) refined science as a systematic pursuit of true knowledge. Aristotle proposed the idea of empiricism, the belief that all knowledge comes into the mind through the senses. In order to create knowledge, the scholar must be able to see, hear, taste, smell, or touch the phenomenon of interest. Aristotle's theory has limitations. Scientists can only observe what they have the tools to observe. Scientists could not observe microorganisms until Antonio van Leeuwenhoek invented the microscope.

Hippocrates of Cos (c. 460–c. 375 BCE) applied Milesian philosophy to Greco-Roman medicine. The Father of Western Medicine encouraged ancient physicians to study their patients' diet and environment. He defined four steps for medical practice: (a) patient examination; (b) diagnosis of disease; (c) forecasting the course of the disease (prognosis); and (d) treatment. The introduction of the scientist-physician was a major shift in the role of the physician and medical treatment. Under the belief that disease was punishment by supernatural beings for sin or lapse of faith, treatments focused on pleasing the gods and goddesses through sacrifices, prayers, and fasting. Physician-caregivers had limited power. Only the gods and goddesses could heal. With the idea that diseases were related to environment, diet, and lifestyle, caregiving focused on active treatment. Physicians gained significance and stature. The shift in power concerned Hippocrates and his followers. Patients were now vulnerable to deception and abuse by unscrupulous physicians. To ensure the dignity and integrity of the medical profession, Hippocrates developed ethical guidelines for medical practice. The Hippocratic Oath is a vow taken by physicians. The oath promises to use medical knowledge to protect life. *Do no harm* is a basic tenet of medical practice and medical research. Physicians may not use their knowledge to intentionally cause injury, pain, or death.

After the fall of the Roman Empire (c. 500 CE), Europe moved into the Middle Ages (c. 1100–1453), a time of disease, famine, and war. People struggled to survive. Science, and certainly the scientific method, seemed irrelevant to daily struggles. The Christian church emerged as the source and gatekeeper of knowledge. The herbal remedies and treatments of ancient civilizations were used but now through the lens of religion. The Christian God determined health and well-being. The idea that the ill or injured person did something to deserve infliction re-emerged. The church promised healing through prayer, piety, sacrifice, or donations. Religious leaders focused on caring for the wealthy and privileged. Secular caregivers, herbalists, and midwives cared for poor people, widows, and the elderly. When the church leaders realized that caregiving engendered power and respect in the community, they labeled the secular healers witches and executed thousands of community caregivers, predominantly females. The church leaders controlled science, education, philosophy, art, and medicine and Europe paid a high price for this control. When the bubonic plague spread to Europe, priest-physicians called people into churches for prayer. Religious ceremonies hastened the spread of communicable disease. In contrast, secular caregivers encouraged patients to rest at home thereby reducing contagion. The Black Death killed almost two-thirds of Europe's population.

The Byzantine Empire of Spain, North Africa, Eastern Europe, and the Middle East thrived during the period known as the Golden Age of Arabic Sciences (c. 800–c. 1200). The Islamic government paid scholars to engage in research and develop ideas to advance society. *The Quran* encouraged Muslim followers to seek knowledge for the sake of knowledge. In Baghdad, the House of Wisdom became a hub of intellectual activity. The House of Wisdom was either a large collection of scholarly works or a community of scholars who shared thoughts, research, and knowledge. Intellectuals from around the world migrated to Baghdad bringing philosophy, literature, art, and inventions from Greece, Rome, Persia, and China. The discovery of paper in China was one of the ideas introduced to the Western world through Baghdad's intellectual community. Before paper, people wrote on animal skins (parchment), thin layers of stone (slate), wood, papyrus, or clay. These materials were heavy, expensive, and difficult to transport. Paper was lighter, more durable, and inexpensive, an ideal way for scholars to share ideas. Mathematics, education, and health care developed from the communication and collaboration of Muslim and global communities. The shared knowledge led to many practical discoveries. Physicist and mathematician Hassan Ibn al-Haytham (c. 966–c. 1039) performed numerous experiments investigating optics, light refraction, and anatomy and physiology of the eye. His systematic method of study earned him the title of the "Father of the Scientific Method." The development of algebra, geometry, trigonometry, and calculus helped identify regular and safe shipping routes for worldly exploration and trade. Knowledge of the human body advanced greatly. Physician Ibn al-Nafis mapped the circulation of blood through the heart and lungs and authored an 80-volume medical encyclopedia documenting medical knowledge. Jabril ibn Bukhtishu and other physicians combined their Christian beliefs of helping others with the medical knowledge of ancient Greeks to create places for caregiving, known as bimaristans. These early hospitals were divided into wards specializing in various diseases. Trained staff provided the latest surgical and medical treatments. No one was denied care for lack of ability to pay. The House of Wisdom ended with the Siege of Baghdad by Hulagu Khan in 1258.

By the end of the Islamic Golden Age, Europe was moving into economic and social recovery. The religious dogma and superstitions of the Middle Ages diminished. Critical thinking, respect for scientific evidence, and rational thought emerged. The Renaissance (c. 1300–c. 1600) brought renewed interest in art, literature, philosophy, and the emerging sciences. As paper became more available, some members of the lower socioeconomic class learned to read. Education, the ability to read, created a group of people who were formerly poor and could now make wise decisions about how to barter their skills and resources. The wealthy no longer held a monopoly on opportunity, wealth, and power. The middle class emerged. The discovery of the printing press by Johannes Gutenberg in 1439 spurred further social changes. The printing press reduced the cost and time of printing. Written information became even less expensive and available to more people. Knowledge was no longer constrained by the church, wealth, and politics. New ideas and philosophies emerged, including Humanism. Humanistic philosophy encouraged respect for individual autonomy and freethinking. The cultural and intellectual movements of the Renaissance transformed the way that people think, who is allowed to think, and what they are allowed to think. The creativity, freethinking, and emerging middle class formed a new foundation for science.

The Scientific Revolution (c. 1550–c. 1700) brought many new discoveries about the universe and nature. Copernicus proposed the heliocentric model of the earth orbiting around the sun. Newton introduced laws of motion and gravitational pull. Anatomists dissected and studied human corpses to advance medicine, anatomy, and physiology. In the process of all of these discoveries, scholars defined and refined the scientific method. Francis Bacon (1561–1626) published *Novum Organum*, or New Method, in 1620. Bacon's work followed Aristotle's empirical approach, proposing that knowledge is gained through seeing, hearing, touching, tasting, or smelling. *Novum Organum* advocated for a systematic approach to experimentation in order to eliminate the influence of personal bias or outside factors. Bacon and French philosopher René Descartes (1596–1650) developed the idea of inductive reasoning. Inductive reasoning is a type of logic that gathers information from individual cases or elements in order to develop theories about a larger, similar group. Bacon and Descartes proposed that scientists could use systematic observations to observe samples and draw conclusions from those cases. Biologists, chemists, physicists, psychologists, sociologists, medical, and public health researchers all use inductive reasoning in their studies. For example, the cancer researcher who studies breast cancer is able to make assumptions about breast cancer by studying a smaller number of cases rather than studying all cases of breast cancer. The inventions, knowledge, and development of various fields during the Scientific Revolution paved the pathway for practical advancements in the modern era. For example, the study of optics for magnification was used to create glasses and the microscope, which enabled scientists to identify and examine microorganisms.

Not all scientific disciplines progressed at the same speed or time. The fields of biology, chemistry, anatomy, physiology, and medicine developed much earlier and more quickly than the field of psychology. Differences in how and when various disciplines developed trace back to the concept of empiricism and what can be observed or derived from the senses. Anatomists could dissect and examine the gastrointestinal system or circulatory system to see how the body works. It is more difficult to examine a living and functioning brain. Much of our knowledge about the brain comes from observing personality and behavioral changes in previously healthy individuals who suffered brain injury due to trauma, stroke, or surgery. Wilhelm Maximillian Wundt (1832–1920) is recognized as the scholar responsible for advancing psychology as a distinct scientific discipline. While training as a physician at the University of Heidelberg, Wundt worked in the physics laboratory studying sense perception and medical psychology. In 1874, Wundt combined his interests to create the first experimental psychology text-book, *Principles of Physiological Psychology*. As professor at the University of Leipzig, Wundt opened the first science laboratory dedicated to psychological research. Wundt's laboratory was a huge success, training many of the world's preeminent psychologists and earning him the title of "Father of Experimental Psychology." Looking back at his achievement, Wundt credited Ernst Heinrich Weber (1795–1878), an earlier professor at the University of Leipzig with carving the path for the famous laboratory. Weber presented psychology as a rigorous science where psychological constructs could be measured and compared for analysis. Wundt was able to build on this idea to develop a laboratory to study the human mind. The emergence of psychology as a unique discipline is an example of how scientists build on the knowledge and function of other scientists, even scientists outside of the discipline to advance an area of interest. New sciences, new disciplines, new fields emerge each year as scientists continue to research, discover, and create.

LIMITATIONS OF THE SCIENTIFIC METHOD

The scientific method is a useful tool. The process offers guidelines for efficient research allowing scientists to discover, investigate, or explore complex problems. However, there are limitations to the process. The scientific method suggests, not mandates steps. There is no policy or law that says scientists must follow the scientific method. Research is considered a creative endeavor, unconstrained by mandatory methods or procedures. Sir Isaac Newton's law of universal gravitation is an example of a discovery that seems to have occurred outside of the scientific method. Newton's biography reports that the physicist first identified gravitational pull while relaxing in an apple orchard. Newton saw an apple fall straight to the ground and realized that there was no curvature to the descent. Although the observation appears accidental, Newton had studied the philosophies of Aristotle and Descartes and was well versed in the current theories of gravity. His observation was not a planned experiment but rather a simple, everyday occurrence during a moment of relaxation. Typically, scientists do not immediately publish extramural observations. They go back to their laboratory, test their observations in an experimental setting, and then announce the discovery to other scientists. The reality is that while the scientific method offers a template for discovery, not all discoveries occur through the scientific method.

A second limitation of the scientific method is that none of the steps substitute for critical thinking. The scientist must read, understand, and evaluate past and current literature on the topic, draw rational conclusions from the work of other scientists, design experiments, and analyze complex data. The scientific method cannot tell the scientist what to study or how to investigate the phenomenon. The researcher must think critically and make wise decisions. A conversation between the Cheshire Cat and Alice in Lewis Carroll's *Alice in Wonderland* captures the predicament of beginning researchers:

Alice: "Would you tell me, please, which way I ought to go from here?"

Cheshire Cat: "That depends a good deal on where you want to get to."

Alice: "I don't much care where—"

Cheshire Cat: "Then it doesn't matter which way you go."

Alice: "—so long as I get SOMEWHERE."

Cheshire Cat: "Oh, you're sure to do that, if only you walk long enough."

There are many different ways to explore health issues. Scientists who are starting out in a particular field must work hard to learn what is already known and what needs to be known next. Prior research helps guide researchers forward. Without the groundwork, new scientists can waste a lot of time and resources. Scientific discoveries do not simply drop out of the air, as Sir Isaac Newton's apple seems to have done. Scientific discoveries are the result of hundreds of hours of hard work, reading, learning, assessing, planning, experimenting, failing, and failing again. And even after an important discovery, scientists must work further to convince others of the value and validity of their discovery. The scientific method allows scientists to search for truth in the natural world. The process does not tell the researcher how to find the truth or what those truths are.

A third limitation is that science can only observe and measure what humans have the ability to measure or compare. While Fracastoro came up with the idea of infectious particles in 1546, his theory could not be confirmed until the microscope was invented. Scientists were unable to identify methods of microbial transmission and sources of contamination until almost two hundred years later. In today's world, science cannot measure beauty or define aesthetics, art, or culture. We know beauty when we see it. However, scientists cannot measure beauty. Additionally, the scientific process cannot weigh moral dilemmas or distinguish between right and wrong or good and bad. Beauty, art, culture and ethics are subjective and cannot be measured objectively.

A final limitation of science, and what much of this book is about, is the strong reliance on honesty and integrity. Professional codes of conduct in research go far beyond the Hippocratic Oath of *Do no harm*. Scientists are human beings, exposed to many interpersonal, political, and religious views. Lifelong values, beliefs, and ways of thinking can skew a study influencing how researchers collect data, analyze results, or draw conclusions. When study results contradict personal beliefs, the scientist is confronted with the dilemma of trusting the eyes, ears, and other senses or betraying lifelong beliefs and values. To ensure the acquisition of true knowledge, scientists must function as neutral observers, disregarding personal opinions, politics, and financial pressures. Scientists must maintain an objective point of view, receptive to new information, ideas, or discoveries. To remain objective, scientists must adhere to high levels of honesty and integrity.

RESEARCH MISCONDUCT AND FRAUD

Each step of the scientific method is vulnerable to fraud or misconduct. Scientists may exhibit bias in selecting past literature to review, planning the study, recruiting participants, data collection, or reporting. Each professional organization and community of scientists has their own definition of research misconduct and actions deemed as misconduct vary widely. Generally, research misconduct is defined as an intentional act of deceit performed within the scope of research activities. Federal government agencies that fund research projects define research misconduct as the "fabrication, falsification or plagiarism in proposing, performing, or reviewing research, or in reporting research results. . . . Research misconduct does not include honest error or differences of opinion" (U.S. Department of Health and Human Services 2005). Misconduct may be active, such as unauthorized use of confidential patient information, relationships with study participants that cross professional and ethical boundaries, changing study protocol based on external pressures, falsifying or "cooking" the research data, excluding data that fails to support the study hypothesis, using ghostwriters, or taking credit for the work of others. The misconduct may also occur as a lie of omission, such as ignoring human participant protections, failing to report a conflict of interest with a commercial product or company, failing to include literature that contradicts the study purpose, or overlooking data that are inconsistent with the research hypothesis. In some cases, it is obvious when the researcher intentionally tries to defraud funders, the public, or other scientists. In many cases, the misconduct is open to question and personal or professional interpretation. A large amount of research misconduct goes undetected. In cases where there is an investigation, investigators must determine whether the alleged misconduct was intended to deceive or merely part of the research process, such as cleaning the data to remove errors in data collection or reporting. Other, more common behaviors that border on misconduct are publishing the same data in multiple publications, sharing authorship credit with someone who did not work on the study, using mismatched research designs, dropping data points, or poor recordkeeping (Martinson, Anderson, and de Vries 2005). The federal government definition of misconduct includes the statement "does not include honest error or differences of opinion." This means that researchers may disagree over what the results mean and just because two scientists disagree does not mean that one scientist engaged in misconduct. Scholarly disagreement is welcomed because disagreements strengthen science by raising alternative theories for further investigation.

How common is research misconduct? The Office of Research Integrity of the Department of Health and Human Services reports investigating between one to fourteen cases per year. In 2002, researchers from the University of Minnesota and HealthPartners Research Foundation randomly surveyed early and mid-career scientists who received National Institute of Health (NIH) research grants (Martinson, Anderson, and de Vries 2005). The survey asked a series of questions related to scientific integrity and misconduct. With 3,247 respondents, the survey became a landmark study in scientific misconduct. The most commonly reported behavior was inadequate record keeping, reported by 27.5 percent of respondents. Fifteen percent of respondents reported dropping data points based on gut reaction. Less commonly reported behaviors were falsifying data (0.3%), ignoring human participant protection requirements (0.3%), and failure to disclose a conflict of interest (0.3%). A later review of multiple surveys on scientific misconduct found that 2 percent of scientists admitted serious research misconduct and 34 percent admitted questionable research practices (Fanelli 2009). When asked about colleagues' misconduct, 14 percent reported misconduct and 72 percent reported questionable research practices (Fanelli 2009). Researchers in medicine and pharmacology reported higher numbers of misconduct than other disciplines. To date, much of the research on misconduct has been through self-reported survey. The main limitation of self-report is that participants are less likely to acknowledge their own misconduct. Despite limitations, the surveys provide some indication of the extent of scientific misconduct.

It is difficult to detect misconduct. Scientists work alone and are not heavily supervised. The systems that exist to prevent or intervene with misconduct are flawed. As noted above, 7 out of 10 scientists report witnessing questionable research practices. The individuals who report misconduct are often dismissed, demeaned, criticized, or rebuked for reporting. In some cases, whistle-blowers are blamed for the fraudulent activities. Few institutions want to admit scientific misconduct within the ranks especially if the scientist is bringing fame and fortune to the institution. Institutional investigations may take months to years. Investigators must prove that the misconduct occurred and was intentional. Once a research study is published, journals are slow to retract articles believing it reflects badly on their own publishing practices. Few journal editors want to admit that they were hoodwinked into publishing faulty or fabricated information. If a scientist is found to have engaged in research misconduct, the consequences range from minor to very serious. The most common outcome is loss of credibility. Peers will question the value of the perpetrator's contributions to the field. True scholars will distance themselves from the alleged perpetrator by neglecting to cite the individual's other publications. Scorned scientists quickly fade from the professional arena. The direct financial consequences of research misconduct relate to future study funding. Scientists rarely fund their own research. In the United States, experiments are supported by state or federal governments, nonprofit organizations, and businesses. The cost of a study can range from a few hundred dollars to millions of dollars. The scientist who accepts funding and then fabricates data takes money under false pretenses and may face fines, dismissal, or imprisonment. There are a few rare cases where the perpetrator was criminally convicted. The challenge is catching the perpetrator in the act and then proving that the deceit was intentional and not human error. Lack of direct supervision, desire by organizations to protect their reputation, and potential for retaliation against whistle-blowers make it easy for corrupt individuals to manipulate the system.

The implications of scientific misconduct on the general public vary by discipline and type of misconduct. In health and medicine, falsified results have implications for science, patient care, and professional practice. Scientists build their research on previous knowledge and studies. Fabricated results mislead other researchers, wasting time and effort on misinformation. Incidents of misconduct damage public trust in science and scientists. Study participants are less likely to volunteer for studies if researchers seem dishonest or corrupt. Integrity is particularly important in health, medicine, and psychology where lives are at stake. For example, if a for-profit business claims that their product will make the consumer look younger or more beautiful and the claims are false, the consumer will lose money, time, and trust in the company. If a pharmaceutical company, a physician, or a psychologist claims that a product effectively treats an illness, more than money is lost. The patient loses valuable time when evidence-based treatments may have been used. During the lapsed time, the disease could worsen or complications may set in.

Scientific misconduct is not a new phenomenon. The Piltdown Man is recognized as one of the biggest frauds in scientific history. In the early 1900s, archaeologists in France, Germany, and Belgium discovered cave drawings, tools, and fossilized remains of early humans. The search for the missing link between man and ape created a sensation around the world. Fueled by strong feelings of nationalism, each country wanted to prove that they were the origin of civilization. Lawyer and amateur archaeologist Charles Dawson was eager for recognition as a full-fledged scientist. Exploring Pleistocene gravel pits near the village of Piltdown, East Sussex, England, Dawson claimed to find a group of skull fragments (and later tools). He contacted Arthur Smith Woodward, a curator at the Natural History Museum, London about his discovery. Smith Woodward joined the search and reconstructed the fragments to reveal a human-like cranium with an apelike jaw. The duo announced their discovery at the Geological Society meeting in 1912. Smith Woodward estimated the Piltdown man to have lived 500,000 years ago. A few scientists questioned the find. The skull was unlike discoveries in Africa, which revealed an apelike cranium with humanlike jaws and teeth. Nevertheless, preeminent scientists, the British press, and the British public embraced the claim for over 40 years. In 1953, the skull was determined to be forgery. The skull pieces were human, stained to look old. The jaw was from an orangutan and the teeth were the fossilized teeth of a chimpanzee. Both men died before the hoax was discovered. During his lifetime, Smith Woodward received numerous awards and recognition for his contributions to paleontology. Dawson is credited with other questionable discoveries, such as a mummified toad encased in rock called "Toad in a hole," a sea serpent in the English Channel, and a new species of fish, a cross between carp and goldfish. Both men enjoyed vast attention and prestige throughout their lifetimes.

Cases of misconduct include some of the biggest names in science history. The Father of Modern Genetics, Gregor Mendel, reported perfect data in his famous study of dominant and recessive traits of pea plants. Too perfect. Statistically improbably perfect. Reviews of the friar's data suggest that he either placed peas with questionable characteristics in the category that supported his hypothesis or failed to count and classify the entire sample of peas (Fisher 1936). Charles Darwin is believed to have plagiarized his theory of evolution from his grandfather, Erasmus Darwin. A review of Louis Pasteur's laboratory notebooks suggests that he exaggerated the success of his rabies vaccine trials. Nobel Prize winning physicist Robert Millikan omitted study results that did not match his desired calculation. Sigmund Freud lied about curing patients with mental illness through psychoanalysis. Educational psychologist Cyril Burt, famous for enumerating the degree of intelligence that is inherited, fabricated results and co-investigators. Some cases of misconduct, such as the Piltdown man, waste valuable time as other scientists examine and debate the results. Other cases, such as Louis Pasteur's rabies vaccination do prove to be true. In his book, *The Great Betrayal: Fraud in Science*, journalist Horace Freeland Judson raises the question: Is an action misconduct if the findings or conclusions are later confirmed to be true?

FORMS OF MISCONDUCT

There are many different types of research misconduct and terms to describe the various behaviors. In 1830, physicist Charles Babbage named and defined four types of scientific misconduct: hoaxing, forging, trimming, and cooking. *Hoaxing* is intentionally tricking someone as either a joke or a prank. Babbage noted that the prankster expects to be discovered. *Forging* is also a form of deception where the forger creates an imitation of the original specimen for the purpose of deception. The forger does not expect to get caught. Forging is now known as fabrication (see Chapter 7 for further description). *Trimming* is the act of adjusting outliers, moving data points that fall very much above or below the mean. During statistical analysis, the researcher might take a score or point that is considered too high and use it to adjust a point that is very low. Trimming is not intended to change the main study results, only to present a picture of a clearer, cleaner set of data. *Cooking* consists of calculating the data differently in order to get the results one wants. As with trimming, the purpose of cooking is to create the image of accurate and precise data. Hoaxing, forging, trimming, and cooking were considered the original types of scientific misconduct. As individuals find new and creative ways to manipulate science, other forms of misconduct emerged and continue to emerge.

Nobel Prize winning chemist Irving Langmuir used the term *pathological science* to describe unintentional self-delusion by scientists. In order to study and understand a phenomenon, one must first believe that the phenomenon exists. With pathological science, the scientist goes through the steps of collecting, analyzing, and reporting data. However, observations are tainted by existing beliefs and expectations. Pathological science is not intentional fraud. Faulty conclusions occur when personal beliefs interfere with the ability to objectively investigate a phenomenon. One example of pathological science is Cachexia Africana or Mal d'Estomac. In the late 1700s, several doctors published cases of dirt eating among slaves in the West Indies and American South (Headen 1837). The cases were described very clearly and scientifically. Sufferers ate clay, chalk, or dirt. Symptoms included pallor, depression, weakness, and difficulty breathing. The disease was noted among African slaves who had "been badly clothed, ill fed, and lodged, and whose constitutions have been worn out by hard labour" (Davidson 1798, 282). Doctors proposed many causes, such as a deficiency of carbon or other essential minerals and failed to mention the most likely causes, starvation, maltreatment, and abuse at the hands of white slave owners. While the doctors noted some degree of relief from warm clothing, a diet that included vegetables and animals, and kinder treatment, the suggested treatment was moving slaves to marshy areas for "hydro-carbonic air." Marshy areas in the South in the 1800s were plagued with mosquitoes carrying malaria. At the time, doctors believed that all people of color were immune to malaria. We now know that carriers of sickle cell trait have some resistance to malaria. Individuals with sickle cell trait would have survived (albeit with a shorter life span due to sickle cell) while individuals without sickle cell would have been at high risk for malaria infection. When a scientist follows the scientific method, it is difficult to discern the influence of potential biases. Pathological science often passes as science because it seems borderline believable, especially if the views are shared by the majority of society. If the pathological bias is intentional, where the scientist is attempting to manipulate data to prove a particular point, sell a product, or gain attention, the body of work meets the definition of research misconduct. If the pathological science is unintentional, the work may be deeply flawed but does not meet the definition of misconduct.

The term *pseudoscience* derives from the words *pseudo* meaning false and *science* meaning knowledge. Pseudoscience is defined as a field, discipline, or set of beliefs that appear to be based in science, yet are not. Examples of pseudoscience include homeopathy, crystal healing, magnet therapy, faith healing, and therapeutic touch. On initial review, reports or reviews appear to be legitimate. Key differences are that pseudoscience tends to be vague in reporting proposed and actual study methods, data analysis, or results. The researcher may use obscure language or hide behind technical jargon. The lack of clarity makes study replication difficult. In reporting the results in conferences or other professional arenas, presenters tend to be evasive. Rather than openly discussing study limitations, the presenters press a particular agenda, typically motivated by financial gain or personal, political, or professional objectives. Questions or criticisms are handled defensively rather than through open exchange of ideas. Pseudoscience is also referred to as junk science, counterfeit science, fake science, or disinformation. Pseudoscience varies from pathological science in that pseudoscience involves intentional deceit by the presenter.

The National Demonstration Project to Reduce Violent Crime is an example of pseudoscience. In 1993, Dr. John Hagelin, chairman of the Department of Physics at Maharishi International University in Fairfield, Iowa, proposed that coordinated and sustained Transcendental Meditation (TM) could establish a field of consciousness capable of creating peace within a community. Hagelin's idea was based on string theory, a concept from physics that proposes that point particles exist as one-dimensional strings exerting influence on other strings. On June 5, 1993, 5,000 TM experts gathered in Washington, D.C., for the *National Demonstration Project to Reduce Violent Crime*. Over the next two weeks, the practitioners silently meditated focused on calming D.C. residents and visitors and reducing violent crime. The exercise gained vast media attention. At the end of the project, police data reported an increase in violent crime. Hagelin responded that the data needed further analysis. A year later, Hagelin released the final project report. The report presented a time-series analysis with the conclusion that violent crime decreased 18 percent during the mass meditation. When questioned about the discrepancy between police crime reports and study findings, Hagelin explained that the data were calculated based on what crime *would have been* without TM and taking into account fluctuations in the earth's magnetic field. No explanation was provided as to how the statisticians enumerated the impact of the earth's magnetic field on violent crime in the city. The appearance of experimental procedures gave the impression of scientific credibility without the depth of explanation.

Plagiarism is a form of misconduct where the writer takes credit for the words or ideas of another person. The action may be intentional, where the plagiarist presents the work as his or her own, or unintentional plagiarism where the plagiarist recalls a phrase or idea and fails to note the original source. Many well-known cases of plagiarism occur in the music industry. The first major case reported in popular music was in 1963 when Chuck Berry's lawyers sued the Beach Boys for copyright infringement. The Beach Boys' song "Surfin' U.S.A." appropriated the tune of Chuck Berry's "Sweet Little Sixteen." The Beach Boys settled the case, listing Chuck Berry as songwriter of "Surfin' U.S.A." Plagiarism, whether it is in music, art, literature, or science, is theft of intellectual property. In science, plagiarism rarely results in legal dispute. Yet, the misconduct is still harmful. The original author loses credit for hard-earned achievement. Failure to receive credit impacts career and future research funding. The person who has had work stolen will also be very cautious in sharing research findings in the future, undermining a basic principle of science. For a field to advance, information must be shared within the scientific community. Failure to share information stymies the discipline. The person who plagiarizes loses because expectations increase. After an important discovery or insight, peers and supervisors expect further groundbreaking discoveries. Unable to deliver, the plagiarist steals more work increasing the possibility of discovery.

Fraud is intentional deception motivated by personal or financial gain. A key part of the definition is intentional. Pathological science may be fraud if the researcher knowingly and intentionally manipulates science to forward a personal or political agenda. If the researcher did not intend to deceive others and was merely attempting to remove inaccurate information, the behavior may not be fraud. Fraudsters may use pseudoscience to cover up the deception. However, not all pseudoscience is fraud. Some people believe strongly in their treatment or intervention and want to share what they consider a good thing with others. Because fraud is about intention, it can be hard to detect. It is difficult to know what is going on in the fraudster's mind. Perpetrators are understandably secretive and privacy may be confused with prudence. Examining the type of environment in which the fraud occurs and the characteristics of perpetrators provides some clues to intent. At the institutional level, fraud occurs more easily and frequently in organizations that are large and complex with poor systems of communication. Top management sets the tone of an organization. If employees see company leaders engage in questionable behavior, corruption, or nepotism, they are more likely to act in similar ways. Poor organizational control and expecting employees to police themselves create opportunities for fraud. Conversely, too much organizational control sets the tone that employees cannot be trusted. Employees will then act on the corporate culture of distrust. Family and intimate partner relationships between coworkers create opportunities for collusion circumventing organizational controls. At the individual level, fraudsters tend to be arrogant, controlling, and have little regard for other people. They are also charming. Their charm is a weapon that both disarms the victim and protects against accusations. The following cases describe two cases of unbelievable fraud, actions, and the personal characteristics of the perpetrators leading to a failure to detect misconduct.

Elizabeth Holmes and Theranos

Elizabeth Holmes withdrew from Stanford University during her sophomore year to start a company with Ramesh "Sunny" Balwani. Theranos, a portmanteau of *therapy* and *diagnosis*, promised to revolutionize the blood testing industry. Without any background or training in biology or medical technology, Holmes and Balwani claimed to invent the *Edison*, an instrument that could run several different laboratory tests from just one small drop of blood. Patients who feared needles or were too busy to schedule medical appointments could walk into a pharmacy and analyze their blood on the spot. The pretty, young, blonde-haired, blue-eyed entrepreneur marketed the company while Balwani managed operations. Holmes's image and defiant story of success without medical training or higher education attracted an impressive list of investors. Within a year, the couple raised six million dollars for their start-up business.

Dr. Ian Gibbons joined Theranos in 2005. With a PhD in Biochemistry from Cambridge University and holding several patents on blood assay techniques from his previous job at Biotrack Laboratories, Gibbons was the first real scientist hired by Theranos. He was responsible for developing blood assay techniques for the Edison. Over time, Gibbons grew increasingly concerned. Results of blood tests analyzed by the Edison did not match results from conventional tests. Analyses by Edison were inconsistent and wildly inaccurate. Gibbons tried to work with company engineers to fix the problems. However, Balwani fostered a climate of paranoia and fear. Corporate culture discouraged communication between departments. Employees who asked questions were warned to stop. When Gibbons pressed for quality improvement, he was accused of having ridiculously high standards. Gibbons's concerns were exacerbated by Holmes's overly zealous and highly effective marketing. By 2010, Holmes raised $92 million in venture capital and had gathered an impressive Board of Directors. The board members were politically and socially affluent, yet had no medical background. While Holmes promised mass production of Edison, Gibbons knew that the instrument was not ready for mass production. Balwani's heavy-handedness made it difficult to address technical problems. In 2013, Gibbons was called to give deposition for a lawsuit between Holmes and a former friend and fellow entrepreneur. Gibbons knew that he would either have to lie under oath or tell the truth. He feared retaliation by corporate executives if he told the truth. The day before he was scheduled for the deposition, Gibbons took an overdose of acetaminophen and wine. He was hospitalized and died a week later from liver failure. By 2015, Theranos was valued at nine billion dollars. Holmes was featured on *Time* magazine's list of the most 100 influential people in the world, *Forbes* list of the most powerful women and *Glamour* magazine's woman of the year. Walgreens, Cleveland Clinic, Capital BlueCross and AmeriHealth Caritas and other large financial backers were eager to collaborate with Theranos. Despite numerous media interviews, Holmes remained secretive about the company. When asked to describe how Edison worked, Holmes never gave a straight answer.

Tyler Shultz had just graduated from Stanford University with a degree in Biology. His grandfather, former Secretary of State George Shultz was on Theranos's Board of Directors. Holmes was a family friend. When Tyler landed a job with the innovative company, he was happy. He was responsible for pilot testing Edison at Walgreens. Within eight months, he noticed problems. Tests were only accurate about 65 percent of the time. Yet, Theranos was reporting results to Walgreens customers. Inaccurate laboratory tests meant that individuals with health problems may not be getting the follow-up care they needed. Shultz suspected that Theranos employees were substituting questionable results with fabricated values. He was hesitant to report his concerns. By now, Holmes and Balwani had surrounded and insulated themselves with very powerful and wealthy people. Shultz eventually reported his concerns and then immediately resigned. Retribution was swift. Balwani called Shultz ignorant and arrogant, lacking a basic understanding of the science behind the instrument. Theranos lawyers threatened him with legal action if he broke the company's nondisclosure agreement. He became estranged from his grandfather who opted to support Holmes. The young man was forced to hire legal counsel to protect his reputation.

In 2014, Pulitzer Prize winning journalist John Carreyrou was investigating fraudulent billing of Medicare. The investigative team revealed misuse and abuse of taxpayer funds in reimbursement for medical office visits, physician self-referrals (when doctors refer patients to a service where they are part owner), and medical testing. Medicare paid for Theranos's questionable laboratory tests. Carreyrou interviewed Shultz and published a scathing report on the company in the *Wall Street Journal*. After the news broke, the Federal Bureau of Investigation (FBI), Securities and Exchange Commission (SEC), Food and Drug Administration (FDA), and Centers for Medicare and Medicaid Services (CMS) investigated Theranos. CMS stopped reimbursement due to problems with equipment, procedures, and training at Theranos laboratories. The FDA ordered Theranos to stop using the Capillary Tube Nanotainer (CTN) because the instrument was not cleared as a Class II medical device and was not approved for interstate commerce. Holmes and Balwani faced charges of fraud. Beyond the financial loss to taxpayers and investors, one million patient laboratory results were invalidated. A million people had been given false test results. Some of these people may have sought treatment when they did not actually need treatment. Others may have delayed intervention not realizing they were at risk for a particular disease that could have been revealed through legitimate testing.

The fact that Holmes and Balwani were able to gather billions of dollars in funding and perpetuate fraud for over a decade is astonishing. The systems and people that should have stopped the deceit failed at almost every level. No one questioned how Holmes was able to develop a complex instrument when she had no background in biology, medicine, or diagnostic technology. Instead, the media embraced the young, charismatic elite college dropout who made big promises and shunned scientific language. Holmes was the antithesis of the stuffy, old, arrogant scientist. No one questioned Balwani's control of the company. The culture of paranoia came across as protection of corporate secrets. The Board of Directors did not own their lack of knowledge and failed in their duty to protect shareholders and customers. The Board functioned as office ornaments and became so immersed and invested in Holmes and Theranos that they refused to listen to whistle-blowers. The system of laboratory test reimbursement and Medicare were too large to properly vet and supervise corporate beneficiaries. There was no application of the scientific method and no internal or external review of Edison. The two people who did try to follow the scientific method left the company, one in a very drastic and horrifying way. The case of Theranos shows how easily unscrupulous individuals can use science to dazzle funders and the media.

Elias A. K. Alsabti, Master Plagiarist

Elias Abdel Kuder Alsabti worked in the cancer research laboratory of Dr. Al-Sayyab while attending Basra Medical College from 1971 to 1974. Before completing medical school, Alsabti reported developing a novel test that could detect certain forms of cancer. Early detection prompts early treatment, reduces medical costs, and decreases premature deaths. The Iraqi healthcare system, a socialized medical system, could benefit socially and financially from early cancer detection. Iraq authorities moved Alsabti to Baghdad and set him up in his own research laboratory, the Al-Baath Specific Protein Reference Unit, named after the Arab Socialist Ba'ath Party. The diagnostic test was named after the president of Iraq, Ahmed Hassan Al-Bakr. The unit's first project was to screen factory employees for cancer. Alsabti charged for the laboratory services even though medical services should have been covered by the national health system. Lab results were never delivered to factory employees. The Iraqi government started investigating and Alsabti immediately went into hiding. Back in Basra, former mentor Al-Sayyab was facing problems of his own. Two drugs that he claimed to treat cancer were found to be ineffective. Al-Sayyab was facing charges of fraud and banned from leaving the county. Alsabti predicted the same consequences. He escaped Iraq and headed for Jordan claiming political persecution.

In Jordan, Alsabti told officials that he had a medical degree and had done groundbreaking research in cancer treatment. He was introduced to the royal family who were impressed by the young man. His Royal Highness Crown Prince Hassan helped Alsabti secure a position at King Hussein's Medical Center in Amman. With the support of the royal family, Alsabti attended international conferences. At one conference in Brussels, Alsabti introduced himself to microbiologist Dr. Herman Friedman of Temple University in Philadelphia. Alsabti told Friedman that the Jordanian government was willing to fund his research assistantship at Friedman's lab. In September 1977, Alsabti showed up at Temple unannounced. He gained a position as an unpaid assistant in the laboratory and enrolled in graduate courses as a non-matriculated student, pending submission of his medical school transcripts. Friedman quickly noticed problems with Alsabti's work. The young scientist did not seem to understand basic laboratory procedures or the pathophysiology of cancer. When the medical school transcripts never arrived, Temple University told Alsabti to drop classes and leave Friedman's laboratory. Within a month, Alsabti made his way across town and gained a position in Dr. E. Frederick Wheelock's laboratory at Jefferson Medical College. Alsabti used the position to enter Jefferson's clinical oncology program and several prestigious medical societies. He claimed he was in a postdoctoral program at Jefferson University. In April, two laboratory colleagues presented Wheelock with evidence that Alsabti was fabricating study data. Wheelock told Alsabti to leave the laboratory. On his way out, Alsabti took several documents, a grant application and research manuscripts. Alsabti later published Wheelock's work as his own. When Wheelock found out and accused Alsabti of plagiarism, Alsabti responded that he had credited Wheelock by including him in the list of references. In his opinion, he had given Wheelock appropriate credit. Wheelock sent letters to *Nature, Science, The Lancet,* and the *Journal of the American Medical Association* encouraging journal editors to check credentials before publication. Only *The Lancet* agreed to publish Wheelock's letter.

By the following September, Alsabti had moved to M.D. Anderson Hospital in Houston. Presenting a letter of reference purportedly from the Surgeon General of Jordan, Alsabti was assigned to work as an unpaid volunteer in Dr. Giora Mavligit's medical laboratory. Between 1977 and 1979, Alsabti churned out dozens of scientific articles. His curriculum vitae (CV) listed 43 articles, a Bachelor of Medicine, Bachelor of Surgery degree and several postdoctoral positions. Some of his papers listed him as completing a PhD. Alsabti's scam was simple. He would take an already published article, replace the author's name with his own name and send the manuscript to a lesser known journal. It was highly unlikely that the original author would ever see the paper. Except one author did. Daniel Wierda was a PhD candidate at the University of Kansas when he saw his manuscript, his future career, published in the *Japanese Journal of Medical Science and Biology.* Wierda's original paper had been sent for peer review to a researcher at M.D. Anderson. Alsabti had stolen the manuscript from the reviewer's mailbox, changed the title, added his own name, and sent it to the international journal. Wierda contacted the journal editors and others with his concerns. Alsabti was asked to leave Mavligit's laboratory. Alsabti eventually applied for and was accepted to medical school at the American University of the Caribbean. He was not required to move to the Caribbean. He could complete his clinical rotations at Houston's South West Memorial Hospital. After completing his medical degree and armed with a CV that listed 60 publications, Alsabti joined the University of Virginia's (UVA) medical residency program.

Alsabti's victims were now working together to gain attention. *Science* published an article describing the plagiarism of Wierda's and Wheelock's articles. UVA officials questioned Alsabti. He gave conflicting responses and eventually resigned from the program. In his one and only media interview, Alsabti claimed that he was the victim. Others had stolen and plagiarized his work. After UVA, Alsabti applied for medical licensure in Arkansas, Nebraska, Washington, and Massachusetts. He worked in Boston, London, Florida, Indiana, and Pennsylvania. Patients called him Dr. Gucci. He was always well dressed, handsome with a wonderful charming bedside manner. In 1989, the Massachusetts Board of Registration in Medicine revoked his medical license after an investigation revealed that Alsabti had plagiarized in order to gain advantage over other candidates. The board concluded that Alsabti lacked the moral character to practice medicine. In 1990, the Associated Press reported that Alsabti died in a car crash in South Africa. An official death certificate was never filed.

The fact that Holmes, Balwani, and Alsabti were able to lie, steal, and cheat so easily highlights weaknesses in the system of checks and balances of science. The primary safeguards against faulty science are peer review and scientific replication. After a discovery, the scientists share their methods and findings at professional conferences and in professional journals. Peers discuss the merits of the findings and limitations of the study. Peer reviewers read and give feedback on research methods and results before publication and dissemination. If the study results do not match the researcher's conclusions, peers will reject the findings and the study. Many studies are denied publication due to faulty methods or questionable results. This system ensures that journals present readers with credible science. The system promotes autonomous regulation by the researcher. The assumption is that individual researchers will act with honesty and integrity because failure to do so will eventually be discovered and draw negative publicity. Replication, where other scientists try to get the same results through similar experiments, is a second safeguard. If the study passes peer review, other scientists will try to replicate the original study. Successful replication confirms the initial findings. Knowing that other scientists will attempt to replicate the study and study results protects against skewed or false research. Other scientists can only achieve the same results if the original study results are true. The process of peer review and replication fosters self-regulation because the scientist should be concerned with getting caught and losing credibility. Despite internal checks and balances, research misconduct is unfortunately, all too frequent. Some experts describe this as the fox guarding the henhouse. Those who stand to gain the most from misconduct are expected to police their own behavior. Furthermore, when questions emerge and investigations do occur, professional journals and organizations want to be discrete fearing that scandals, misprints, or journal retractions could tarnish the reputation of the publisher and undermine public confidence in the discipline. The scientific method is highly vulnerable to manipulation and fraud. Grant funders, peer reviewers, journal editors, other scientists, and the general public have important roles to ensure that scientists follow the scientific method with integrity and honesty.

FURTHER READING

Davidson, G. 1798. "Account of the Cachexia Africana: A Disease Incidental, to Negro Slaves Lately Imported, into the West-Indies." *Medical Repository* 2 (3): 282–84.

Fanelli, Daniele. 2009. "How Many Scientists Fabricate and Falsify Research? A Systematic Review and Meta-Analysis of Survey Data." *PLoS ONE* 4 (5): 1–11.

Fisher, R. A. 1936. "Has Mendel's Work Been Rediscovered?" *Annals of Science* 1 (2): 115–37.

Gower, Barry. 2002. *Scientific Method: A Historical and Philosophical Introduction*. New York: Routledge.

Headen, B. F. 1837. "Cachexia Africana." *Western Medical Reformer* 2 (July): 290–94.

Judson, Horace Freeland. 2004. *The Great Betrayal: Fraud in Science*. Orlando, FL: Harcourt.

Magner, Lois N. 1992. *A History of Medicine*. New York: Marcel Dekker.

Martinson, Brian C., Melissa S. Anderson, and Raymond de Vries. 2005. "Scientists Behaving Badly." *Nature* 435 (7043): 737–38.

Mendoza, Abraham O. 2011. "Resolution and Composition—The Beginnings of the Scientific Method." *World History Encyclopedia, Credo Reference: Academic Core*. Accessed December 16, 2019. https://search-ebscohost -com.ezproxy.sju.edu/login.aspx?direct=true&db=edsgvr&AN=edsgcl .2458802534&site=eds-live

Miller, David J., and Michel Hersen. 1992. *Research Fraud in the Behavioral and Biomedical Sciences*. New York: Wiley.

National Institutes of Health. 2010. "Research Integrity." Accessed May 5, 2018. https://grants.nih.gov/grants/research_integrity/research_misconduct .htm

Suvajdžić, Ljiljana, Aleksandra Djendić, Vladimir Sakač, Grozdana Čanak, and Dragan Dankuc. 2016. "Hippocrates—The Father of Modern Medicine." *Vojnosanitetski Pregled: Military Medical & Pharmaceutical Journal of Serbia* 73 (12): 1181–86.

University of Texas Arlington. *Finding Quantitative and Qualitative Research: Distinguishing Article Type.* Accessed June 1, 2018. http://libguides.uta .edu/researchtype/evaluating

U.S. Department of Health and Human Services. 2005. "Federal Register: 42 CFR Part 93." Accessed June 1, 2018. https://ori.hhs.gov/sites/default /files/42_cfr_parts_50_and_93_2005.pdf

TWO

Human Participant Protections

Information is power. Anytime someone collects information about another person, no matter how trivial or benign the information seems, the person taking the information gains authority over the subject of the information. Health information is particularly vulnerable to creating power imbalance because health and social history may reveal weaknesses about the subject of the information. The information may be used to harm, manipulate, or control the other person. Individuals lose jobs, insurance coverage, friends, and reputation when diseases or behaviors with negative social stigma are shared with employers, family members, or community members. To protect human study participants from abuse of power, medical research is guided by ethical principles. Ethics define appropriate behavior. Ethical principles trace back to the earliest civilizations. In order to survive, early humans and their ancestors, hominins, formed social groups. Group members shared responsibilities of hunting, fishing, gathering plants, meal preparation, childcare, and protection. Over time, norms and rules developed to define expectations of behavior within the community. Without such rules, the group could not function. Individuals would not have been able to trust one another, and the community would have broken down. Some rules became laws. For example, it is illegal to steal from, harm, or kill someone. Ethics are broader than laws and suggest—not mandate—how to behave. One ethical principle is the Golden Rule of *do unto others as you would have them do unto you*. The Golden Rule encompasses the values of kindness, respect, and consideration for others. Most people learn moral values as children through fairy tales, stories, or modeling of behavior by parents, grandparents, teachers, and other influential adults. Some values are learned in adulthood through work or interpersonal relationships. Universal ethical principles, values common to communities and cultures throughout the world, are honesty, integrity, loyalty, justice, respect for others, accountability, and trustworthiness.

Ethics are important to professional groups because they create a culture of competency by suggesting acceptable behaviors, practices, and boundaries. Each professional group has their own set of guiding ethical principles. Ethical principles of psychologists, medical doctors, sociologists, and educators typically encompass the universal ethical principles as well as other conventions. Scientists also have ethical guidelines. Research ethics suggest how researchers should behave when studying a topic, collecting data, reporting results, and generally interacting with others. The main ethical principles of science relate to collaboration with other scientists or professionals; potential conflicts of interest; data collection, storing, and sharing; human participant protections; peer review of colleague's research; and dissemination and publication of study findings. The previous chapter presented examples of ethical misconduct related to the scientific method, and later chapters present examples of misconduct during the specific stages of the research process. This chapter focuses on the ethics of protecting human participants in research. Violations of fellow human beings are a most egregious form of scientific misconduct. The principle of *do no harm* or *nonmaleficence* is a basic and timeless philosophy, derived from the Hippocratic Oath. In medicine, *do no harm* means that health professionals should not use their knowledge to cause injury or death to a person. In research, *do no harm* means that the scientist must not intentionally injure study participants in the name of science. Scientists are obligated to put the health and welfare of their study participants above their quest for knowledge. As with early social groups, ethical guidelines in research evolved over time. Many principles developed from cases of intentional or unintentional neglect or malice by scientists.

THE NUREMBERG CODE (1947)

History offers many unfortunate cases where scientists lost sight of the principle of do no harm. During World War II, Nazi scientists performed horrific experiments. From testing the effects of extremes in temperature on the human body to subjecting people to deadly diseases in order to test vaccines, Nazi researchers tortured, poisoned, and killed thousands of people in the name of science. Dr. Josef Mengele was one of several noteworthy characters. Mengele was a rising star in the German scientific community. Handsome, intelligent, and born into a nouveau riche Catholic family, Mengele began his career from a place of privilege. He earned his PhD working with world-renowned biologist and geneticist Dr. Otmar Freiherr von Verschuer at the Anthropological Institute at the University of Munich. As a student, Mengele measured the jaw shape and size of various ethnic groups. His interest in genetic differences continued with his medical thesis, *Genealogical Studies in the Cases of Cleft Lip-Jaw-Palate*. Reviewers note that these early studies of investigating physical differences of ethnic groups were consistent with genetic science of the time (Weindling 2004).

At the age of 20, Mengele joined the anti-Semitic paramilitary Stahlhelm (Steel Helmet), progressing to the Sturmabteilung (SA) and eventually Schutzstaffel (SS). He rose quickly through the ranks. By the time Mengele assigned to the concentration camp Auschwitz, he was a well-respected physician-scientist, SS officer, and decorated war hero. Mengele enjoyed ultimate authority over all Auschwitz prisoners, his study subjects, and peers. As concentration detainees arrived on trains, he stood tall and handsome on the platform and decided who would go directly to the gas chambers, who would go to the forced labor camps, and who would become subjects in his experiments. Mothers hoped their children would be chosen by Mengele. He appeared so handsome and kind. He even brought the imprisoned children candy and other goodies. Mengele's experiments soon deteriorated into physical abuse, lethal injections, and murder. One study injected dye into the eyes in an attempt to change eye color. He dissected body after body, operating on subjects without anesthesia. Although some historians suggest that the studies were intended to forward the Nazi agenda of creating a pure Aryan race, Mengele's activities went beyond eugenics. He was a cold, calculated killer, harvesting brains and other tissue specimens for his adviser, Verschuer. Mengele preferred twin experiments. He would expose one twin to a toxic or harmful procedure. When the subject died, he would kill the other twin to autopsy the body and look at anatomical differences between the two siblings. Over one million people were killed at Auschwitz. An estimated 3,000 twins plus thousands of other study subjects died in Mengele's laboratory. His experiments lacked any scientific basis. Although Mengele worked constantly, his work yielded no new knowledge or scientific benefit. Records indicate that he collected volumes of data without any final analysis. There is no record of reports to professional groups or in scientific journals.

Victims of the German concentration camps had no choice in study participation. Their bodies were used as human petri dishes without consent or regard to study procedure or outcome. After the war, 23 doctors and administrators, including Mengele, were tried for war crimes and crimes against humanity. Seven of the defendants were acquitted, seven were sentenced to death by hanging, and the remaining were sentenced to prison for terms ranging from 10 years to life in prison. The Nuremberg court indicted Mengele. However, he was never brought to justice. After the war, Mengele was captured and held as a prisoner of war. The American army released him, not realizing he was a notorious criminal. With the help of his wealthy family, Mengele escaped to South America. The Nuremberg Code was established in 1947 to address the atrocities found by the War Crimes Trials. The basic tenets of the Nuremberg Code are:

- Scientists must be trained in scientific procedures.
- Animal testing should be done before testing on humans.
- The study must be reasonable and justifiable based on prior research.

- The research must yield benefit to society.
- Participants must voluntarily and freely consent to study procedures.
- Participants are free to withdraw from the study at any time.
- Facilities must be adequate to prevent harm or injury.
- The researcher must not inflict unnecessary harm on participants.
- The researcher should stop the study if the procedures are found to be dangerous.

The Nuremberg Code is a set of guidelines for biomedical research. It is not law.

THE DECLARATION OF HELSINKI (1964)

Twenty of the 23 defendants in the Nuremberg Trials were physicians. This spurred the World Medical Association (WMA) to develop a statement reminding physicians of the Hippocratic Oath and professional obligation to care for patients. The Declaration of Helsinki started with the Declaration of Geneva. The Declaration of Geneva encourages respect for the autonomy and well-being of patients and warns doctors not to use their medical knowledge to harm or violate human rights. The Declaration of Helsinki, also by the WMA, defines the basic rights of human participants in biomedical research. Drawing from the Nuremberg Code, the original version of the Declaration of Helsinki asserts the principles of respect for persons; the right to self-determination; the right of the participant to make informed decisions regarding study participation; and if the participant is unable to make an informed decision due to age or mental infirmity, then a parent or legal guardian most be consulted to give consent on behalf of the participant. The document emphasizes that the researcher's primary duty is to study the participant. Participant welfare takes precedence over every other aspect of the study. (Chapter 5 presents cases where the researchers lost sight of their responsibility as doctor first and researcher second. See Dr. Mani Pavuluri and Dr. Albert Kligman.)

Since the original list of guidelines, the Declaration of Helsinki has undergone several revisions. The first revision in 1975 introduced the idea of ethics committees or Institutional Review Boards (IRBs). The fourth revision in 1996 developed as the result of the AIDS Clinical Trials Group (ACTG) Study. Funded by the U.S. Centers for Disease Control and Prevention, the ACTG study was an international study of 477 pregnant women comparing rates of maternal to infant transmission of human immunodeficiency virus (HIV) with the antiviral drug zidovudine. In comparison to placebo, zidovudine reduced transmission by about 68 percent (Connor et al. 1994). The study raised concerns in that study participants living outside of the United States did not have the same access to zidovudine as study participants in the United States. The WMA revised guidelines requiring studies conducted in developing countries be conducted under the same ethical guidelines as the country of sponsorship. The Declaration of Helsinki continues to be debated and revised. Some government agencies recognize the document, while others do not.

TUSKEGEE SYPHILIS STUDY (1932–1972)

Among U.S. researchers, the Tuskegee Syphilis Study is widely recognized as the longest running research study violating the rights of human study participants. Funded by the federal government, the study began in 1926 with the intention of treating syphilis among rural residents in the southeastern states. Syphilis is a nasty disease. Without treatment, the bacteria attack the brain, spinal cord, heart, and other internal organs, resulting in blindness, dementia, muscle paralysis, and death. The microbe *Treponema pallidum* can be transmitted from mother to fetus, causing premature birth, low birth weight, or stillbirth. To convene the study of syphilis, the U.S. Public Health Service (USPHS) partnered with the Julius Rosenwald Fund. The fund was a philanthropy established by one of the business partners of Sears, Roebuck and Company. The Rosenwald Fund provided start-up resources to local school districts to build and sustain schools for African American students who were blocked from attending segregated white schools. The foundation supported over 5,000 schools through a system of matched funding with local school districts. The syphilis study was set up in a similar way in that local and state health departments had to match funding for syphilis treatment within the local community.

The first stage of the study identified prevalence of syphilis in six counties. Nationwide, the prevalence of syphilis was 4.05 cases per 1,000 people, 4.0 cases per 1,000 among white adults, and 7.2 cases per 1,000 among African American adults. Rosenwald's Syphilis Control Survey found 195 cases per 1,000 people. The highest rates were in Macon County, Alabama, with 360 cases per 1,000 people. There are a number of reasons for such high rates. Macon County was geographically and economically isolated from social and medical services. The majority of residents descended from slaves and eked out a living on small tracts of degraded agricultural land. Many had never seen a doctor and relied on home remedies for ailments. The same factors that created high rates of syphilis in Macon County also made the area perfect for a controlled research study. Macon County residents were isolated from outside influences. The plan for syphilis treatment derailed in October 1929 when the stock market crashed and the nation entered the Great Depression. The Rosenwald Fund continued to support the syphilis study; however, local and state public health departments could no longer meet the matched funding requirement.

In 1932, USPHS officials decided to continue the study as a longitudinal study, monitoring men with and without syphilis in Macon County. Officials based the research at the Tuskegee Institute, a historically black college founded by Booker T. Washington. A few treatments were given, often in a haphazard way and not to any extent that would kill the bacteria or halt infection. The treatments at that time were not completely effective. Some study participants were given aspirin or vitamins as treatment. At least one young public health doctor raised concerns regarding the ethics of the study. His concerns were dismissed by officials at the highest echelons of the USPHS. By World War II, penicillin was commercially available as an effective treatment for syphilis. Rather than treating the infected men, the study administrators made the conscious decision to block treatment. USPHS doctors sent lists of study participants to local doctors and asked them not to treat the study participants. The local doctors were so enamored by the idea of working with highly respected government doctors that they did not question the consequences of untreated syphilis in the community. A list of participants was also sent to the Department of Defense (DoD) to prevent the men from being screened and drafted to war. If the men were drafted, the DoD would have done a mandatory physical exam, discovered syphilis, and administered treatment. The DoD agreed not to draft or treat the men on the list.

USPHS officials enjoyed unequivocal authority over local doctors, Macon County public health staff, administrators at the Tuskegee Institute, and the poverty-stricken study participants. Few people dared to question the merits of the study. In 1968, USPHS social worker and epidemiologist Peter Buxton came across reports of the syphilis study. He filed a protest with the Division of Venereal Diseases. Syphilis was a treatable disease. Allowing people to go untreated was unethical. When his concerns were dismissed, Buxton leaked the story to the press. An article reporting the study appeared on the front page of the *Washington Post*. The USPHS had clearly violated the principle of do no harm as well as the basic tenets of the Nuremberg Code. Public outcry and congressional investigation brought the project to a halt in 1972. Over the course of the study, 100 participants died of advanced syphilis. The impact on families and loved ones was beyond measure. The federal government settled a class action lawsuit for $10 million plus the cost of medical care for the surviving men and their wives, widows, and offspring. On May 16, 1997, President Clinton officially apologized to the survivors on behalf of the nation. The racism and abuse perpetrated in the Tuskegee Syphilis Study continues to engender distrust toward doctors, health professionals, and researchers by African American patients.

WILLOWBROOK HEPATITIS STUDIES (1955–1970)

During the early twentieth century, children and adults with physical or intellectual disabilities were separated from society and sent to live in private or state institutions. In some cases, parents could not afford to care for a disabled child and abandoned the child to be cared for by the state. In other cases, families believed that specially trained staff at state institutions could do a better job of caring for their child than they could. To researchers, institutionalized children were an easy supply of study participants. Located on Staten Island, New York City, Willowbrook State School was home for children with disabilities. The school could house up to 4,000 residents. As demand for services increased and funding decreased, the school became dirty, overcrowded, and rundown. Infections, and particularly hepatitis, spread easily throughout these institutions. Hepatitis virus is a highly contagious organism that can survive on a contaminated instrument or surface for over a week. The virus attacks the liver, impairing the body's ability to metabolize carbohydrates, proteins, and fats and to filter toxins from the blood. Most children admitted to Willowbrook were infected with hepatitis within the first year of arrival.

In 1955, New York University School of Medicine pediatrician Saul Krugman partnered with Yale School of Medicine virologist Robert Wayne McCollum Jr. to study hepatitis. Krugman believed that he could create immunity by injecting gamma globulin antibodies extracted from the serum of hepatitis patients into uninfected individuals. Willowbrook was the perfect study site. The studies were approved by New York Department of Health and funded by the Office of the Surgeon General and the U.S. Army. Study participants were housed in a separate unit on Willowbrook grounds to ensure that they were not exposed to other communicable diseases that might interfere with their ability to fight infection. The research ward was clean and well staffed. Parents gave consent for their children's participation. The experimental group was injected with hepatitis antibodies, while children in the control group did not receive antibodies. The study team observed the children over time and monitored rates of hepatitis in the two groups. By 1964, Willowbrook was overcrowded, housing almost 6,000 residents. The main school stopped accepting admissions. However, the research unit still had beds, and administrators referred potential residents and their families to the research unit. Parents who wanted to get their children into Willowbrook had little choice but to sign their children into the study. The hepatitis studies continued to evolve. In later studies, Krugman injected all newly admitted children with antibodies. This means that all new study participants were deliberately exposed to hepatitis. The studies ended in 1970 as advocates for disabled children were investigating the general living conditions at Willowbrook. The school officially closed in 1987.

Krugman's hepatitis studies led to several important discoveries. He discovered that Hepatitis A and Hepatitis B are distinctly different diseases. Hepatitis A is spread by fecal-oral route, while Hepatitis B is spread through blood and body secretions. Krugman was awarded the Robert Koch Prize for excellence in biomedical sciences and the prestigious Mary Woodward Lasker Public Service Award. Despite accolades, the Willowbrook studies are considered one of the most unethical experiments ever performed on children. Defending the actions of the researchers, some scholars point out that the Willowbrook hepatitis and the USPHS syphilis experiments happened during a different era, a time when doctors and scientists were held in high prestige and patients, family members, and study participants were grateful for any care or attention they received. Other scholars raise questions about the basic study methods and Willowbrook management. Why did the scientists opt to test viral hepatitis on children and not the staff who were also exposed to hepatitis while working at Willowbrook? Why did school administrators choose to refer new admissions to the research unit instead of cleaning and sanitizing the main school? How much autonomy did parents actually have in placing their children in the studies? How did Krugman justify intentionally infecting children with a deadly virus? The researchers violated several principles of the Nuremberg Code: the study must be reasonable and justifiable based on prior research; participants must voluntarily and freely consent to study procedures; participants are free to withdraw from the study at any time; the researcher must not inflict unnecessary harm to participants; and the researcher should stop the study if the methods are found to be dangerous. The Willowbrook studies raised the idea of the need for additional research protections for children and other vulnerable institutionalized populations.

MILGRAM'S CONDITIONS OF AUTHORITY (1961–1963)

During the Holocaust, Stanley Milgram's family listened intently to radio broadcasts, hoping for news of family members living in Hungary and Romania. After the war, Milgram and his brother recalled visitors with concentration camp tattoos. The descriptions of suffering and persecution left a lasting impression. Milgram wondered how humans could intentionally hurt other humans. After completing his doctorate in social psychology at Harvard University, Milgram decided to investigate the explanation given by many German officers that they were only "following orders." The popular opinion in the United States was that German people were more obedient to authority than other nationalities. Americans believed that they were independent thinkers and would never allow the atrocities of Nazi Germany to occur in the United States. Working at Yale University, Milgram designed an experiment to explore the topic. How far would the ordinary person go in hurting another person when ordered to do so by an authority figure? The study recruited men of ages 20–50 from the New Haven area. The experiments were conducted at the Yale Interaction Laboratory. As study volunteers entered the laboratory, they were greeted by a scientist and introduced to a second person identified as another study participant. The participants were told that they were taking part in an experiment on learning. Each participant drew a straw to see who would be the teacher and who would be the student. The straws were fixed. The teacher role was always assigned to the New Haven volunteer. The second person was an actor conspiring with the researchers. After drawing straws, the scientist took both men into a room where the learner-actor was seated and strapped to a chair. Electrodes were attached to one wrist, and the learner-actor was given a list of word pairs to memorize. The teacher-study volunteer was then taken to an adjoining room and seated in front of an electrical generator. The machine had a dial with 30 notches ranging from 15 volts (mild shock) to 450 volts (severe shock). The scientist instructed the teacher-study volunteer to administer increasingly higher electric shocks if the learner gave an incorrect response. No electrical shocks were actually given. However, the actor cried or screamed giving the appearance of pain from an electrical shock. If the teacher-study volunteer refused to administer the shocks, the scientist prodded him with scripted statements. All of the teacher-study volunteers administered shocks up to 300 volts. Two-thirds of participants gave shocks up to 450 volts. At the end of the study, participants were debriefed and assured that they had not inflicted harm. Milgram conducted 18 variations of the obedience to authority study changing the location, adding a teaching assistant so that the teacher did not administer the shocks but instead directed the assistant to administer shocks, and a number of other procedural alterations to check his theory.

Based on the experiments, Milgram developed Agency Theory, the idea that in social situations, individuals exhibit either agentic state or autonomous state. In agentic state, the individual allows others to direct his or her actions. In autonomous state, the individual exhibits free will and takes responsibility for personal action. Milgram's Agency Theory applies to many different social situations, such as workplaces, warfare, and bullying. Despite groundbreaking psychological research, Milgram was denied tenure. The study raised ethical concerns about the mental harm done to the study participants and violation of the principle of do no harm. Milgram believed that the criticisms were most likely due to his results. His colleagues, American professors, wanted to believe that Americans had greater autonomy and free thought than Germans. Milgram disproved their opinion and showed that when people are confronted with the decision of hurting another person or refusing to comply with authority, the majority of people will inflict harm. Milgram's study of obedience to authority has been replicated in many places throughout the world with similar results. Approximately 65 percent of people will go against their moral values to please an authority figure.

From an ethical perspective, Milgram's work is an example of how research can also cause moral injury or emotional harm. The theory of Milgram's conditions of authority shows how research assistants may perform harmful procedures that violate human participant protections because they are directed to do so by people in positions of authority. This theme arose repeatedly during the Tuskegee Syphilis Study. Over the four decades of the study, many medical students, doctors, nurses, and USPHS staff were involved with data collection. Very few raised questions about the ethics of not treating syphilis.

THE BELMONT REPORT (1979)

As multiple cases of abuse of study participants and particularly abuse of vulnerable populations came out in the media, people demanded action. Politicians prompted the federal government to develop guidelines for federally funded research. A Presidential Commission was established. The outcome of this working group was *The Belmont Report*. Published in 1979, *The Belmont Report* defines three ethical principles in research: respect for persons, beneficence, and justice. Respect for persons means that study participants are autonomous agents and have the freedom to decide whether they wish to participate in a research study and the freedom to withdraw from a study at any time without suffering injury or retaliation. Beneficence extends the Hippocratic principle of "do no harm" to "do good" or to act with kindness. Justice means that all participants are treated fairly and have equal access to study benefits and risks. One group should not carry the risks of an experiment while another group receives the benefits.

The Belmont Report serves as the basis for the U.S. federal regulations protecting human research participants, known as Title 45 Code of Federal Regulations Part 46. The regulations apply to all research involving humans with the exception of some types of research in schools or other educational settings. Exclusions are (1) research intended to study the effectiveness of educational techniques; (2) tests or surveys where participants are anonymous; (3) public observation of behavior; (4) existing documents, such as historical records; (5) laboratory specimens or diagnostic procedures; (6) research studying social or public benefit programs; and (7) food quality or consumer acceptance studies. Note that the federal regulations still use the term *subject* to refer to people who take part in research studies. In practice, most disciplines replace the term "subject" with "participant" to reflect the fact that study participants are autonomous and not subordinate to the scientists. The federal government continues to update Title 45 Code of Federal Regulations Part 46 as new forms of technology and research emerge. The Common Rule is the policy approved by 17 federal agencies regarding human participant protections. The rule defines requirements for compliance of human participant protections by research institutions, informed consent, and the functions and role of Institutional Review Boards (IRBs).

The main responsibility for human participant protection rests on the primary investigator. However, IRBs work with the researcher to review the study protocol and provide suggestions to ensure protection of human participants. The IRB is a formal committee composed of scientists and nonscientists. IRB members review all research involving humans at institutions that receive any type of funding from the federal government. Studies on laboratory animals are reviewed by an Institutional Animal Care and Use Committee. The IRB members ensure that a study follows the guidelines of Title 45 Code of Federal Regulations Part 46. To complete an IRB review, the primary investigator submits a package of forms to the IRB prior to the start of a study. The forms include a description of the study, study recruitment materials, informed consent documents, and any survey instruments or other related study documents. The study protocol explains why the study is important, how study participants will be selected and recruited, how data will be collected and analyzed, and how study participants will be protected from possible risks or harm. IRB members give feedback on the protocol and study materials, focusing exclusively on human participant protections. It is not the IRB's responsibility to suggest other ways to study the topic or whether they agree with the premise of the study. The review focuses exclusively on whether the primary investigator is following ethical principles to protect human study participants. Once a study is approved by the IRB, the scientist cannot deviate from the proposed plan. While the researcher is responsible for adhering to ethical guidelines in day-to-day procedures, the IRB is responsible for oversight. If a study participant suffers harm during the study, the scientist must decide, with the help of the IRB, whether the study should continue. Unfortunately, many scientists become too involved or too invested in their study and lose sight of the fact that it is easier to stop and revise a study than it is to undo harm to a study participant. The IRB can provide an objective perspective pointing out potential pitfalls in study methods and interactions with study participants.

RESPONSIBILITIES OF THE RESEARCHER

Over time, best practices in human participant protections ethics continue to develop. The primary investigator, the main scientist, is responsible for ensuring that study volunteers are protected from harm throughout the study procedures and in reporting results. Responsibilities of the primary investigator are to ensure that:

- All members of the study team are qualified to perform study procedures and complete regular training in human participant protections.
- The study is scientifically sound and based on current knowledge in the field.
- The study is designed to yield legitimate results.
- Selection of study participants is clearly defined and that all volunteers meet the eligibility criteria.
- The study is approved by an IRB and carried out according to the study protocol.

- Study volunteers or their legal guardians are given full disclosure concerning the nature of the study, study procedures, and alternatives to study participation.
- Participant identity is protected by maintaining anonymous or confidential procedures in data collection and reporting.
- Participant rights and well-being are monitored throughout the study.
- Any adverse events are reported to the IRB and other relevant authorities.

The researcher must consider human participant protections at every step of the scientific method, from identifying a problem to study through final data collection and reporting. Any form of scientific misconduct violates the researcher's responsibility for human participant protections. For example, the scientist who engages in pathological science violates human participant protections by wasting the time and energy of study participants in an experiment that does not advance knowledge. The Tuskegee Syphilis Study lacked such a scientific foundation. The doctors believed that syphilis progression varied by color of skin. There was and is no scientific evidence to support this theory.

One important component of human participant protections is *informed consent*. The concept of informed consent arose from the Nuremberg Code, the idea that study participants should be autonomous, free to determine whether they wish to take part in a study. Informed consent consists of two parts: informed and consent. *Informed* means that the researcher must fully disclose the nature of the study, procedures, risks, benefits, and alternatives to the experimental treatment to the study participant. Information must be communicated in a language or dialect that is easily comprehendible to the study participant. Some IRBs recommend no higher than seventh or eighth grade reading level. Since the Common Rule requires researchers to include 18 different elements in the consent form, it is often difficult to meet the reading-level requirement. Reviews of consent forms suggest many are at the tenth grade reading level (Larson, Foe, and Lally 2015). If the study participant's mental capacity to understand study procedures or study purpose is limited due to age or mental deficits, consent must be obtained from the legal guardian acting in the best interest of the study participant. *Consent* means that the study participant voluntarily agrees to take part in the study and is not acting under coercion. Reflecting back on the Tuskegee Syphilis Study, the men were coerced to participate in the study in that they were told that they were receiving treatment for "bad blood," a slang term for syphilis. They also received small tokens, such as rides in a car (a prestigious experience for poor farmers), medical exams, and funeral expenses. Mothers who gave their children to Dr. Josef Mengele believed that they had no other choice. In practice, either verbal or written consent is collected at the start of the study. However, informed consent does not end with the act of consent. The researcher is responsible for updating participants if new information emerges that may influence someone's decision to participate. One way to understand informed consent is to view the study participant as a partner in the research study, a partner who is investing time and resources throughout the study procedures. In research, children, prisoners, institutionalized people, and pregnant women are considered vulnerable populations. Vulnerable populations require special protections under the code of federal regulations. The researcher must take extra precautions to ensure that harm does not come to study participants in the category of vulnerable populations.

It is the researcher's responsibility to know, understand, and adhere to responsible research. If a study participant experiences an adverse event during the study, the researcher must review study procedures and determine whether the adverse event is the direct result of the study. If the event does appear to be related to the study or study procedures, the researcher must contact the IRB and decide whether to stop or modify the study. The main focus of any study is always on those who are volunteering to help scientists explore human nature.

THE PSYCHOANALYTIC STUDY OF THE CHILD (1953–1997)

In 1916, many young, single pregnant women were shamed into giving up their babies for adoption. Thousands of minority children became wards of the state, destined to grow up in state-run orphanages. Philanthropist Louise Waterman Wise founded the Child Adoption Agency of the Free Synagogue in New York City to match Jewish orphans with adoptive families. After World War II, the Free Synagogue agency was renamed Louise Wise Services serving a wider population of children and families. Dr. Viola Bernard (1907–1998) was a highly respected social psychiatrist and child welfare advocate who served on the board of Louise Wise Services for 50 years. In her capacity as chief psychiatric consultant, Bernard wielded considerable influence in agency operations. Working with the founder's daughter, Bernard formalized adoption procedures and expanded services to children of color. Under Bernard's direction, the agency established the Interracial Adoption Program and the Indian Adoption Project. (In 1978, Congress passed the Indian Child Welfare Act protecting Native American children from forced removal and adoption by nonnative families.) Bernard believed that twins raised together placed a strain on adoptive parents and thwarted each child's ability to develop a unique identity. Although there was and is no evidence to support the idea, Bernard advocated for separating twins and triplets at adoption and not telling the adoptive parents that there were other siblings. She believed that knowledge of the sibling interfered with parent-child bonding. Because of the stigma of illegitimacy, adoptive parents rarely asked about the biological mother or possible siblings.

Dr. Peter Neubauer was a board member with Louise Wise Services, director of the Jewish Board of Guardian's Child Development Center, and clinical professor of psychiatry at New York University. He heard of Bernard's intention to separate twins at birth and realized the potential for a unique study. Most twin studies were retrospective, asking the twins to recall past experiences. Retrospective studies are limited by what the participant remembers. A prospective study, a study that followed separated monozygotic siblings over time, could record less memorable experiences and explore the question of nature versus nurture. Neubauer envisioned a prospective study comparing the influence of genetics, social environment, and parenting practices. Bernard agreed to serve as coinvestigator on the project. Five sets of twins and one set of triplets were enrolled in the study. Thirteen families were carefully selected based on the presence of an older sibling in the home and age, socioeconomic status, educational level, and religion of the parents. The presence of an older sibling, also adopted from Louise Wise Agency, ensured that parental demographics were known by the researchers, and the parents already trusted agency officials. Infants were intentionally placed with dissimilar families. For example, one of the triplets was placed with a blue-collar family, a second with a middle-class family, and the third with a wealthy family. Study personnel were advised to keep the fact that the child was from a multiparous birth "confidential." This is misuse of the term *confidential*. In research, the term "confidential" means not telling people outside of the study the identity of the study participants. It does not mean keeping information from the study participants themselves. To explain data collections, adoptive parents were told that their infant was part of The Psychoanalytic Study of the Child, an ongoing study of child development requiring annual home visits and psychological testing. The name of the study did not betray the fact that the children were from multiparous births. The study was managed by the Jewish Board of Guardians Child Development Center and partially funded by the National Institute of Mental Health. Data were collected every three months over the first year, every six months throughout ages one to three years, and then every year until the child reached around nine years of age. Data measurements consisted of IQ, personality assessments, eye-hand coordination, and inkblot images. Children were filmed to document characteristic mannerisms and physical and cognitive development. Neubauer was not actively involved with the study. Staff later recalled a disorganized study with lots of data (Perlman and Segal 2005). Interestingly, when Neubauer approached the Catholic adoption services agency to expand the study, the director, Sister Bernard, responded that what God has created should not be torn asunder and refused to separate twins or triplets.

The secret research began to unravel in 1980 when one study participant, Robert Shafran attended Sullivan County College in New York. Classmates mistook Shafran for Edward Galland, a student who had previously attended Sullivan County College and decided not to return. Stunned by the amazing similarities, a current student introduced Shafran to Galland. The families immediately recognized the young men as birth brothers. David Kellman saw news stories of the Shafran-Galland reunion and immediately noticed the physical resemblance between himself and the young men. Kellman contacted Galland's mother and learned that all three shared the same birthday and were adopted through Louise Wise Services. The story of the separated and then reunited triplets was a media sensation. The brothers appeared on talk radio, movies, and television shows. When the triplet's adoptive parents met with Louise Wise Services, demanding to know why the brothers were separated, the agency explained that it was too difficult to find one adoptive family for triplets. Mr. Kellman immediately responded that he would have adopted all three boys. Louise Wise administrators stuck to their explanation, and the families left with their questions unanswered. However, when one of the fathers returned to the conference room to retrieve his umbrella, he found the agency administrators opening a bottle of champagne. News of the separations helped to reunite some of the other siblings. Critics of the separations noted how the twins and triplets were deprived of the opportunity to share childhood experiences and adventures. They would never know the social connections that could or should have been if they had been allowed to grow up in the same family. In 1980, New York made it illegal to separate twins at birth.

Some journalists exaggerated the details of the study to create a more riveting story. Several journalists reported that the siblings were separated specifically for the experiment, rather than by the adoption agency. One source reported up to 21 sets of twins and triplets participated in the study. The research remains clouded in secrecy and mystery. Neubauer never published the full results of the study and refused interviews citing clinical reasons. He claimed the information would be harmful to the siblings. When Neubauer died, he left The Psychoanalytic Study of the Child documents to Yale University Library. The documents, labelled Manuscript Group 1585, are sealed until October 25, 2065, and may only be opened with permission of the Jewish Board of Children's Family Services. The library inventory only lists records of 11 children. With authorization, the triplet brothers were able to obtain some documents related to their data. They reported that the documents were heavily redacted and difficult to understand. Viola Bernard left her papers to Columbia University on the condition they remain sealed until 2021. Columbia is considering extending the seal until 2065 for consistency with the Neubauer papers.

In limited interviews, Neubauer offered the explanation that informed consent was not common when the study started. By today's standards, The Psychoanalytic Study of the Child study presents multiple human participant protections concerns. The researchers never considered the possibility that the siblings might meet each other. It was assumed that the biological mothers were "young, unwed, and promiscuous" and that adoptive parents and the children would never want to know the biological mother or the circumstances of the child's birth (Perlman and Segal 2005, 272). With the internet, facial recognition, and DNA matching programs, it is easier for genetically similar family members to find each other. Today's researchers must consider the short- and long-term implications of a study. A second issue is that the study did not just look at genetics. It looked at the interaction of the child and the environment. The adoptive parents and siblings were just as much a part of the study as the children. The researchers examined parenting practices and social demographics. They even interviewed the older siblings. Yet the parents were never informed that they were also study participants.

CONFLICT OF INTEREST

A conflict of interest occurs when a person must fill two roles and the responsibilities and expectations of one role compete with the expectations of the other role. Bernard held dual roles as child psychologist for Louise Wise Services and researcher in The Psychoanalytic Study of the Child. Conflicts of interest are common in business, law, government, finance industry, and research. In the case of Theranos (described in chapter 1), board members were both financial supervisors and close friends of Holmes. They held two simultaneous roles. Dual roles are common in medical research because industry and pharmaceutical companies fund many research studies. Many advancements could not be made without such partnerships. When Alexander Fleming discovered a mold that dissolved the cell walls of bacteria, he and other researchers struggled to create enough of the substance for experiments. Collaboration with several large pharmaceutical companies allowed large-scale extraction, production, and clinical testing to make the antibiotic penicillin a medical reality. The National Institutes of Health National Center for Advancing Translational Sciences, President's Council of Advisors on Science and Technology, Wellcome Trust, World Economic Forum, Gates Foundation, and the Food and Drug Administration (FDA) encourage partnerships between academic institutions, scientists, and industry.

In medical research, health professionals have a professional responsibility to do no harm, to act in the study participant's best interest. However, researchers are also employees, contracted to work for a company and to act in the company's best interest. Betraying corporate interest could mean loss of job, study funding, or even one's career in research. The presence of a conflict of interest does not automatically mean that an individual must act inappropriately betraying one responsibility. In many cases, the conflict of interest can simply exist and the individual must consider and negotiate dual responsibilities on a case-by-case basis. Full disclosure, informing everyone involved about the conflict of interest, is one way to prevent or negotiate potential conflict. On the other hand, some scientists are hesitant to disclose a conflict of interest, claiming that such disclosure creates unwarranted skepticism. Readers will not trust the research or the researcher who accepts payment from a company with financial stake in the study results.

Problems occur when one set of responsibilities corrupts the other set. A scientist may manipulate study design, data collection, statistical analysis, or participant interaction when consultancy fees or research funding is on the line. However, motivation for corruption is not always financial. Corruption may occur when social, personal, or career aspirations conflict with professional obligations. In the Tuskegee Syphilis Study, local doctors were corrupted by the opportunity to network with high-level government doctors. They overlooked the potential harm of not treating syphilis and betrayed their professional role as physicians. Corruption does not have to be intentional. The actor may not even realize he has devolved into corruption. He may lie to himself and justify the actions. The Comparison of Atypicals in First Episode Study shows how dual roles and conflict of interest can have fatal consequences in medical research.

Comparison of Atypicals in First Episode Study (2002–2015)

In March 2002, AstraZeneca started the Comparison of Atypicals in First Episode (CAFE) Study. The 52-week double-blind study compared three FDA-approved antipsychotic medications, commonly referred to as *atypicals*. The market for this new class of drugs was growing exponentially. AstraZeneca hoped to show that their drug was superior to atypicals manufactured by other pharmaceutical companies. The CAFE study was managed by Quintiles, a contract research organization (CRO). The Department of Psychiatry at the University of Minnesota served as one of 26 study sites. Under terms of the contract, AstraZeneca paid the Department of Psychiatry $15,648 per participant who completed the study. Initially, University of Minnesota researchers struggled to fill the study, and Quintiles placed the department on probation. In April 2003, the Department of Psychiatry opened Station 12, a special psychiatric inpatient unit at Fairview University Medical Center. Every patient admitted to Station 12 was evaluated for study participation. Within eight months, the department enrolled 12 patients and was recognized by Quintiles for turning their poor performance around.

The purpose of the CAFE study was to compare the effectiveness and side effects of Seroquel (quietiapine, manufactured by AstraZeneca), Zyprexa (olanzapine, manufactured by Eli Lilly), and Risperdal (risperidone, manufactured by Janssen Pharmaceuticals) among patients who were experiencing their first psychotic episode (Keefe et al. 2007). Psychosis is a symptom of mental illness. The first episode of psychosis is characterized by hallucinations, seeing, hearing, or believing things that are not real, delusions of special powers, or important missions directed by supernatural beings. Patients in psychosis have trouble thinking clearly and will say and do things they would not normally do. Under the AstraZeneca study protocol, participants were randomly assigned to one of the atypical drugs. The patient could not come off the drug for the duration of the study, even if the treatment was not working or the patient was experiencing adverse effects. The study protocol excluded suicidal participants. It did not exclude participants who were homicidal. The study only compared atypicals. It did not compare older antipsychotic medications, such as Trilafon (perphenazine) or Haldol (haloperidol). AstraZeneca may have excluded the older antipsychotic medications because pharmaceutical companies were making a fortune off the newer drugs and previous studies suggested that the atypicals were no better than the older drugs. There was no financial benefit to including the older established drugs in the clinical trial.

One of the patients admitted to Station 12 was Dan Markingson. Dan graduated from the University of Michigan in 2000 with a degree in English and moved to Los Angeles with the goal of becoming a screenwriter. While visiting Dan, his mother, Mary Weiss, noticed bizarre behaviors. Dan had changed his last name and repeatedly asked her about a mysterious upcoming event. Mary had no idea what the event was. In his apartment, Dan had encircled his bed with candles, wooden posts, and money. He claimed the objects protected him from evil spirits. When Markingson became extremely agitated, Weiss called the police. The police dismissed her concerns as overreaction. Over the next several months, Markingson's psychotic behaviors worsened to include homicidal ideations. He told Mary that he was taking direction from a group called the Illuminati. In November, Markingson visited his mother in Minnesota. He told her that he would kill her if the Illuminati instructed him to do so. On November 12, 2003, Markingson threatened to slit his mother's throat. Weiss called emergency medical services. Markingson was taken to a Saint Paul hospital and later transferred to Station 12 under the care of Dr. Stephen C. Olson, associate professor in psychiatry at the University of Minnesota.

On November 14, Markingson was deemed mentally incompetent. Olson recommended involuntary commitment, and the decision was confirmed by a second clinician. Under the terms of commitment, Markingson could avoid involuntary hospitalization by agreeing to follow Olson's treatment plan and consenting to regular follow-up. On November 21, Jean Kenney, the study coordinator at Station 12, asked Markingson to participate in the CAFE study. Kenney had previously had difficulty enrolling patients when their parents or guardians objected to the study. She was careful to ask Markingson when his mother was not around. When Weiss found out, she was upset. How could Dan be simultaneously competent to agree to study participation and mentally incompetent to care for himself? Dr. Olson and Station 12 staff dismissed Weiss's concerns. On December 8, Markingson was discharged to an outpatient facility under the condition that he follow Olson's treatment regimen. Over the next several months, Markingson continued to struggle mentally. Weiss and Markingson's social workers reported an angry, isolated, and withdrawn individual who expressed ideas of grandiosity and delusions. Weiss wrote five lengthy letters to Olson and the study team, expressing concerns for her son's condition. Olson responded that the atypical was working and Markingson's condition was improving. On May 8, 2004, Dan Markingson used a box cutter to slice open his abdomen and nearly decapitate himself. He was found dead in the bathroom of the outpatient facility.

When the study blind was lifted, Weiss learned that Markingson was on AstraZeneca's drug, Seroquel. Over the course of the study, AstraZeneca had paid $327,000 to the University of Minnesota. By 2008, Seroquel was one of the nation's most profitable drugs with sales reaching almost $4 billion. Mary filed several official complaints against the university, Olson, and others. The FDA investigated the case and found no significant violations of research protocol or federal regulations. The Minnesota Office of the Legislative Auditor (2015) investigated and identified multiple ethical violations. The key findings of the auditor's report were that:

- The researchers took advantage of Markingson's impaired mental state in asking him to consent to the study. They did not have a patient advocate present when Dan signed the consent form even though the IRB protocol stated that each patient would have an independent advocate.

- Markingson was coerced into following the experimental treatment plan because the alternative would have been involuntary commitment to inpatient care.

- Olson had a financial incentive to keep Markingson in the study. AstraZeneca only paid per patient completing the study. If Markingson dropped out or required a change in medication, AstraZeneca would not pay.

- The study team ignored or dismissed Weiss's concerns and complaints regarding her son's symptoms and condition.

- Jean Kenney performed tasks beyond her scope of practice as a licensed social worker.

- The University of Minnesota's IRB failed to perform a thorough review of an adverse event. When the IRB was made aware of the suicide, they only interviewed Olson and neglected to review Markingson's medical records to determine whether the suicide was related to study participation.

- The expert consultant hired by the Minnesota Board of Medical Practice to investigate complaints against Olson had multiple conflicts of interest. The expert was a faculty member in the same department as Olson, shared space in the Ambulatory Research Center where the CAFE study took place, received more than $83,000 from AstraZeneca in 2006, and chaired the university's IRB. Despite multiple connections to Olson, the Department of Psychiatry, and AstraZeneca, the consultant assured the medical board that he could remain impartial in his investigation.

- The University of Minnesota Board of Regents failed to respond appropriately to Markingson's death. The explanation given was that the university was a $3.5 billion organization with 23,000 faculty and staff. Discussion of individual cases of concern would be "impractical and unwieldy" (Office of the Legislative Auditor 2015, 27).

The state auditor suspended all drug studies by the University of Minnesota Department of Psychiatry and recommended legislation to monitor patients in psychiatric drug studies at the university. The case of Dan Markingson raises the issue of how well individuals and organizations can monitor and police themselves to care for study participants, especially when large amounts of money are at stake. Bioethicist Frederick Grinnell (2014) estimates $5,000 is the price tag for research integrity. When a researcher received $5,000 or more, ethics violations are more likely to occur.

ETHICS DUMPING

The need for research into global health problems creates the potential for exploitation of human study participants in countries without resources to support human participant protections. *Ethics dumping* is the exportation of unethical research practices to low- and middle-income countries by researchers in high-income countries (Schroeder et al. 2018). There are two types of ethics dumping. The first type is when the researcher does research that would be considered exploitive in the high-income country. The second type is when the researcher or the host country disregards or does not understand ethical guidelines for research practice. Human participant protections may be neglected due to insufficient resources to support an ethics committee, lack of expertise of committee members, failure to empower the committee, pressure from sponsors, or pressure from the researcher.

Genetic Research in Anhui, China

Anhui is one of China's poorest provinces. Residents are isolated by poverty, geography, and limited public transportation. As a result, the genetic makeup of the people of Anhui is unusually homogeneous. The large, uniform gene pool is ideal for investigating genetic deviations. In 1994, Harvard professor Geoffrey Duyk partnered with Scott Weiss and Xu Xiping. Duyk was planning to leave Harvard to join Millennium Pharmaceuticals, a biotech start-up. Weiss was an epidemiologist with expertise in respiratory diseases. Xiping was a recent gradu-ate of Harvard and was originally from the Anhui district. With local connec-tions, Xiping could influence and mobilize the collection of blood from this unique and highly valuable gene pool. Millennium agreed to pay $3 million for the blood samples of Anhui residents (Pomfret and Nelson 2000). The pool would provide samples for multiple pharmaceutical research projects. Astra AB (now AstraZeneca) paid $53 million to investigate respiratory disease within the sam-ple. Hoffmann-LaRoche invested $70 million for obesity and diabetes research related to the Anhui blood samples. Public offering of Millennium Pharmaceuti-cals on the stock exchange raised another $54 million.

In 1996, Xiping was named director of Harvard's Program for Population Genetics. He established a network of academics from Anhui Medical University and local public officials to collect blood samples from local residents. The regional health director was named co-investigator of the project. Residents, many illiterate, were promised $10 per day to cover food and travel. In exchange for the blood sample, they would receive free medical exam, test results, and follow-up care. Local government officials pressured reluctant citizens through a strategy known as *thought work*. Within the communist society, very few resisted. Over 16,600 people donated blood to the Harvard genetic bank. The researchers never fulfilled their end of the bargain. The researchers never delivered test results. Study participants were paid $1.50–$3.00 per day for blood donation. The cards promising free or reduced treatment were worthless. Patients were never provided with care. Residents lost trust in doctors and local health officials.

Chinese journalists investigated complaints by the local people and found that the research had not been approved by a Chinese ethics committee, some resi-dents were not aware that they were taking part in a research study, and study participants were never given informed consent. In 1999, Harvard sent a team to investigate complaints. The team found no concerns with the research. Several months later, the Department of Health and Human Services (DHHS) launched an investigation, spurred by whistle blower Gwendolyn Zahner, a former Harvard School of Public Health faculty member. The DHHS investigation found proce-dural errors in supervision and record keeping. However, there was no evidence to support the accusation that study participants had been harmed. In 2003, the Chinese Ministry of Health issued regulations restricting the export of special medical resources. In 2008, Takeda Pharmaceutical Company purchased Millen-nium Pharmaceuticals for $8.8 billion. Senior executives earned millions of dol-lars in stock trades.

Ethical principles developed as a way to safeguard society. In research involv-ing human participants, the principles of beneficence, justice, and respect are timeless principles designed to safeguard the welfare of human study partici-pants. While the primary responsibility for ethical experimentation is on the researcher, the IRB and government agencies provide oversight to ensure human participant protections are honored. A drawback of ethical principles is that individuals are conditioned to believe that other members of society, including scientists, will act with honesty and integrity. Unfortunately, this is not always the case. Some people believe that they do not have to live by the same rules as other people. This may be due to arrogance, racism, sexism, ableism or other form of authoritarianism that creates a misguided perception of inequality and allows one to take advantage of others. Later chapters present further cases where conflict of interest or poor practices interfere with good science. Chapter 9, "Solutions," discusses systems and best practices to ensure that every researcher is personally responsible for protecting the people who volunteer their time and effort to support science.

FURTHER READING

Abrams, S. 1986. "Disposition and the Environment." *The Psychoanalytic Study of the Child* 41: 41–60.

Barry, M. 1988. "Ethical Considerations of Human Investigation in Developing Countries: The AIDS Dilemma." *The New England Journal of Medicine* 319 (16): 1083–86.

Connor, E. M., R. S. Sperling, R. Gelber, P. Kiselev, G. Scott, M. J. O'Sullivan, R. VanDyke, et al. 1994. "Reduction of Maternal-Infant Transmission of Human Immunodeficiency Virus Type 1 with Zidovudine Treatment. Pediatric AIDS Clinical Trials Group Protocol 076 Study Group." *The New England Journal of Medicine* 331 (18): 1173–80.

Drazen, Jeffrey M. 2015. "Revisiting the Commercial–Academic Interface." *The New England Journal of Medicine* 372 (19) (May 7): 1853–54.

European Commission. n.d. "Ethics." Accessed June 1, 2019. https://ec.europa.eu /programmes/horizon2020/en/h2020-section/ethics

Grinnell, Frederick. 2014. "The Interrelationship between Research Integrity, Conflict of Interest, and the Research Environment." *Journal of Microbiology & Biology Education* 15 (2): 162–64.

Jones, J. H. 1981. *Bad Blood: The Tuskegee Syphilis Experiment*. New York: Free Press; London: Collier Macmillan.

Keefe, Richard S. E., John A. Sweeney, Hongbin Gu, Robert M. Hamer, Diana O. Perkins, Joseph P. McEvoy, and Jeffrey A. Lieberman. 2007. "Effects of Olanzapine, Quetiapine, and Risperidone on Neurocognitive Function in Early Psychosis: A Randomized, Double-Blind 52-Week Comparison." *The American Journal of Psychiatry* 164 (7): 1061–71.

Larson, Elaine, Gabriella Foe, and Rachel Lally. 2015. "Reading Level and Length of Written Research Consent Forms." *Clinical and Translational Science* 8 (4): 355–56.

Lifton, Robert Jay. 1986. *The Nazi Doctors: Medical Killing and the Psychology of Genocide*. New York: Basic Books.

Lo, Bernard, (U.S.) Institute of Medicine, and Marilyn J. Field. 2009. *Conflict of Interest in Medical Research, Education, and Practice*. Washington, D.C.: National Academies Press. Accessed January 24, 2018. https://www.ncbi.nlm.nih.gov/books/NBK22926/

Loder, Elizabeth, Catherine Brizzell, and Fiona Godlee. 2015. "Revisiting the Commercial-Academic Interface in Medical Journals." *British Medical Journal* 350. http://dx.doi.org/10.1136/bmj.h2957

National Commission for the Protection of Human Subjects of Biomedical and Behavioral Research. 1979. *The Belmont Report*. Washington, D.C.: Office of Human Research Protections. Accessed May 5, 2018. https://www.hhs.gov/ohrp/regulations-and-policy/belmont-report/index.html

National Institute of Health. 2016. "Protecting Human Research Participants." Accessed August 28, 2018. https://phrp.nihtraining.com/codes/02_codes.php

Office for Human Research Protections. 2016. "The Belmont Report." Accessed August 28, 2018. https://www.hhs.gov/ohrp/regulations-and-policy/belmont-report/index.html

Office of the Legislative Auditor. 2015. "A Clinical Drug Study at the University of Minnesota Department of Psychiatry: The Dan Markingson Case." March 19. Accessed November 10, 2019. https://www.auditor.leg.state.mn.us/sreview/markingson.pdf

Perlman, Lawrence M., and Nancy L. Segal. 2005. "Memories of the Child Development Center Study of Adopted Monozygotic Twins Reared Apart: An Unfulfilled Promise." *Twin Research and Human Genetics: The Official Journal of the International Society for Twin Studies* 8 (3): 271–81.

Pomfret, John, and Deborah Nelson. 2000. "An Isolated Region's Genetic Mother Lode." *Washington Post*, December 20. Accessed November 10, 2019. https://www.washingtonpost.com/wp-dyn/content/article/2008/10/01/AR2008100101158.html

Resnick, David B. 2015. "What Is Ethics in Research & Why Is It Important?" National Institute of Environmental Sciences. Accessed June 12, 2018. https://www.niehs.nih.gov/research/resources/bioethics/whatis/index.cfm

Resnick, David B. 2017. "Research Ethics Timeline (1932–Present)." National Institutes of Health. Accessed November 10, 2019. https://www.niehs.nih.gov/research/resources/bioethics/timeline/index.cfm

Schroeder, Doris, Julie Cook, François Hirsch, Solveig Fenet, and Vacantha Muthuswamy, eds. 2018. "Ethics Dumping: Case Studies from North-South

Research Collaborations." Springer Open. Accessed November 10, 2019. https://link.springer.com/book/10.1007/978-3-319-64731-9

Shamoo, Adil E., and David B. Resnik. 2009. *Responsible Conduct of Research*. New York: Oxford University Press.

Weindling, Paul. 2004. "The Ethical Legacy of Nazi Medical War Crimes: Origins, Human Experiments, and International Justice." In *A Companion to Genethics*, edited by Justine Burley and John Harris. Oxford: Blackwell.

THREE

The Literature Review

Scientific study is similar to a work of art. Instead of creating a sculpture or painting, the scientist builds knowledge. Science is an intellectual creation established through incremental and shared knowledge. The path to discovery requires disciplined reading and review of the work of other scientists. In his inaugural address to students, faculty, and administrators at the opening of the Faculté des Sciences of the University of Lille in 1854, microbiologist Louis Pasteur said, "In the fields of observation, chance favors only the mind which is prepared" (Pearce 1912). Pasteur was referring to physicist Hans Christian Ørsted's discovery of electricity and magnetism. During a lecture demonstration, Ørsted noticed the needle of a navigational compass deflect slightly away from the magnetic north. The cause of the movement was a magnetic charge emitted from nearby live wires. The audience did not notice any movement. Ørsted noticed it because he had been studying magnetic fields for 20 years. Just like Newton's observation of gravity based on an apple falling from a tree limb, Ørsted was able to notice something that others did not. He continued to investigate the phenomenon and eventually discovered a new branch of physics. The idea that discovery favors the prepared mind is seen repeatedly throughout history. Microbiologist Alexander Fleming discovered penicillin when he returned to his laboratory after a long vacation and found that his culture of *Staphylococcus aureus* was destroyed by mold samples. Biochemist Karl Paul Link discovered the blood thinner warfarin when a farmer asked Link to investigate why his cows were hemorrhaging and dying. Engineer Wilson Greatbatch was building an instrument to record heart rhythm when he assembled the parts backward. Instead of detecting an impulse, the machine produced an impulse. With refinement, Greatbatch's instrument became the first implantable cardiac pacemaker. These scientists realized each of their discoveries, not by chance, but because of their rigorous intellectual preparation. Researchers invest an enormous amount of time and energy in reading and learning about a problem before initiating an experiment. The literature review informs the researcher on what is known about the issue and what needs to be known in order for the field to advance.

Health problems tend to be complex and impossible to address through one study alone. The first step of the scientific method is defining the research topic by seeing what other scholars have written and found about the issue. These past studies form the foundation for future study. Each study builds on previous knowledge, and together they create the body of knowledge. Researchers wishing to investigate a particular topic start by examining what other researchers have found or surmised about the topic. The literature review shows whether other scientists are working on the topic and if so, current facts and strategies of investigation. The scientist is then able to plan a new study based on previous knowledge. This process ensures that time and resources yield true benefit and avoid wasting time and resources on creating ideas or inventions that already exist.

To perform a literature review, the researcher reads books and research articles, attends professional conference presentations, and reviews other scholarly resources on the topic of interest. As the researcher reads the resources, information is collected on the strengths and weaknesses of previous studies, gaps in knowledge, suggested study methods, possible study instruments, applicable models or theories, and future directions required to advance the body of knowledge. Performing a literature review is very tedious and time-consuming. There are no shortcuts. However, the benefits of a rigorous literature review are incredible. The scientist can ensure that the new study moves the field forward, making a mark in science and humanity. After reading and reviewing existing information, the researcher writes a review of the literature. The written literature review appears at the beginning of an experimental report, after the abstract. The literature review report follows a standard format starting with general information on the topic and gradually narrowing the focus to one specific aspect of the topic. This format helps the researcher to develop one or more focused research hypotheses or research questions and to create a logical, functional study. Problems occur when the researcher skips over the literature review, ignores or discounts previous literature, manipulates the literature to forward an agenda, or uses information from questionable resources.

STATEMENT OF THE PROBLEM

The literature review defines the problem and informs the reader of who, what, where, when and how society is impacted. General information on the extent of the problem, numbers of people impacted, specific populations at risk, protective or risk factors, and health and social consequences of the problem are presented as background to the problem, also known as the *statement of the problem*. The first step of health research is defining the health or social issue. Definitions may be straightforward or may be challenging. Whenever there is an existing definition of a disease or health condition, researchers attempt to use the existing definition. Consistency in definition of the problem ensures that scientists can compare results between studies, strengthening the body of literature on the topic. For example, if a researcher plans to study binge drinking, it makes sense to use the same definition as other experts. The National Institute on Alcohol Abuse and Alcoholism (NIAAA) defines binge drinking as a pattern of alcohol consumption resulting in a blood alcohol concentration (BAC) of 0.08 grams percent or higher. Males typically reach 0.08 BAC by drinking five or more drinks within two hours. Females typically reach 0.08 BAC by drinking four or more drinks within two hours. When studies do not allow for immediate blood monitoring, researchers define binge drinking as five or more drinks for males and four or more drinks for females within a short period. By using this definition consistently, researchers can compare binge drinking among different age groups, genders, years, geographic regions, or other variables of interest. Diagnostic manuals, professional organizations, and validated surveys are all good sources of definitions for health problems.

In some cases, there may not be a definition of the health topic or there is not much literature on the topic. When the problem is new, relatively unstudied, or affects a small number of people and little has been done to investigate the issue, it may be difficult to find scholarly information on the topic. In this case, scientists *benchmark* to similar areas. Benchmarking is a strategy used in business to compare a product, process, or work flow to best practices. One example of benchmarking in health research involved a group of health administrators at Johns Hopkins Hospital (OR Manager 2007). The administrators were concerned with long wait times experienced by patients moving through surgical procedures. The managers wanted to improve patient flow and reduce waiting time. They decided to investigate best practices of companies recognized for efficiency in moving large volumes of valuable packages. Rather than looking at other hospitals, they looked to FedEx and Walmart. Administrators toured the FedEx logistics center in Memphis and Walmart's distribution center in Bentonville, Arkansas. New practices emerged to support safe staffing levels, maintain access to adequate surgical supplies, and promote communication of potential delays in the operating room schedule. Even though the hospital administrators were not actually looking at organizations that moved people, they gained ideas on how to serve patients more quickly and effectively. Benchmarking is a valuable strategy in studying novel problems or as a new way to look at old problems.

MISGUIDED KNOWLEDGE AND EXPERIMENTATION

Experiments lacking scholarly foundation are not actually science. The horrific human experiments by Nazi scientists are an extreme example of what happens when individuals do not base activities on existing knowledge. Physicians and prisoners of Auschwitz described Mengele's research as garbage and the doctor as an arrogant megalomaniac "possessed by pseudoscience" (Lifton 1986, 368). Mengele never published his results. He never produced any novel discoveries. Without a scientific foundation, without novel information that advanced the body of knowledge, experimental procedures are not science. Science is an intellectual activity.

The Tuskegee Syphilis Study is another example of research based on flawed logic. When public health doctors and researchers started the Tuskegee Syphilis Study, medical practitioners already knew the effects of untreated syphilis on the human body. Syphilis had been active in Europe since the late fifteenth century. Dr. Caesar Boeck of the University of Oslo had published a large longitudinal study of 2,000 white European patients with untreated syphilis. U.S. doctors believed there were physiological differences between people with light skin and people with dark skin. Tuskegee doctors thought that syphilis attacked the bones and the heart in African Americans and the nervous system in whites. There was no scientific evidence to support this theory. Moreover, even if there were physiological difference based on skin color, the study design did not account for such a discovery. In order to prove differences by race, scientists would have to compare people of different races. Tuskegee Syphilis Study participants were all African Americans. Whites were not included in the study. The research hypothesis of the Tuskegee Syphilis Study was based on racism.

When experts present biased or racist information as fact, science is held back and people suffer. For over 100 years, doctors believed that women were not at risk for heart disease. Pre-eminent physician, Sir Richard Quain described differences in heart disease as:

> Enlargement of the heart, one of the most distressing and fatal diseases, is more than twice as frequent in males as in females, the precise proportion being 8 to 3. This remarkable liability to enlargement of men's hearts, as compared to those of women, is, he [Quain] thinks, unquestionably due to the greater amount of work and anxiety which, under the present dispensation, falls upon men. Ladies may take this fact to heart, and reflect whether, in claiming the rights of women, they may not at the same time incur the risks of men, and with them a new and unexpected form of disability. They might do wisely to rest content for their sex, with hearts suffering, it may be, from those tender affections which often pain, but never kill. (Influence of Sex on Heart-Disease 1872, 347)

We do not know where Quain got his statistic of 8 to 3. We do know that misconceptions of heart disease as a male problem continued throughout much of the twentieth century. In 1973, a study by Health Insurance Plan of Greater New York began with the statement, "The relatively low incidence of coronary heart disease (CHD) among women in comparison with men is well-known" (Weinblatt, Shapiro, and Frank 1973, 577). The Framingham Heart Study was the first to acknowledge heart disease as an equal opportunity disease. Even then, attitudes were slow to change. Innumerable mothers, wives, and sisters complaining of symptoms of heart attack were dismissed by healthcare providers and sent home to suffer subsequent, often fatal, heart attacks. In terms of science, research into heart disease among women was a missed opportunity. Today, many women still do not recognize heart disease as the leading cause of female deaths because the well-known classic symptom of heart attack, crushing chest pain, is based on studies of men. If women report chest discomfort, it tends to be moderate. For women, the symptoms of heart attack appear as nausea or vomiting, abdominal discomfort, neck, jaw, shoulder, or upper back pain, sweating, lightheadedness or fatigue. Because women do not recognize the signs of heart attack and the possibility of sudden death, many do not seek emergency treatment. The number of women who died and continue to die prematurely due to undetected heart disease is staggering. Basing science, knowledge, and professional practice on skewed logic is dangerous.

REVIEWING PAST RESEARCH

The second part of the written literature review examines existing research studies on the topic. The scientist reviews landmark studies and other recent research. Landmark studies are research studies that yield important insights or discoveries. The Framingham Heart Study is a landmark study in heart disease research. The study provided many new insights into the causes of heart disease and at risk individuals. In reviewing past research, the scientist collects valuable information on how other scientists studied the issue, notes limitations of current studies, and identifies gaps in the body of knowledge. The researcher may also describe and apply relevant models or theories. Models or theories are particularly valuable in research because they can be used as the basis for new studies.

A common mistake by inexperienced researchers is confusing an annotated bibliography with the literature review. An annotated bibliography lists individual sources followed by a short summary paragraph noting facts, opportunities, strengths, or limitations of each source. Researchers use the annotated bibliography format as they gather references. The list helps them to view the different resources and content prior to writing the literature review. An annotated bibliography does not replace the literature review. The literature review outline condenses or combines studies and presents important content information whereas the annotated bibliography may leave gaps in content information. Substituting the annotated bibliography for the literature review places the responsibility for intellectual activity on the reader as opposed to the scientist-author. Writing a literature review requires critical thinking and evaluation of the research to date. A solid literature review is one of the most challenging steps to a research study.

The last part of the written literature review presents what needs to be done next to expand the body of knowledge. This section should proceed naturally from the section reviewing past research studies. If the researcher determines that a particular concept needs further study, then it is logical that the proposed study investigates that concept. For example, if there is not a lot of information on how many people are impacted by a problem, the researcher may want to investigate incidence or prevalence. Health research often follows standard disease management practice. The typical order of addressing an emerging health issue is: (a) define the problem, (b) identify who is affected, (c) determine effective treatment or intervention, and (d) identify how to prevent the problem. The first step is for scientists to develop a case definition of the problem. Defining the problem includes describing the disease, signs and symptoms, and related diagnostic or laboratory tests. Once a case definition is established, studies seek to determine the extent of the problem, numbers of people affected, social or economic cost, health consequences, and common complications. Incidence or prevalence rates identify at risk populations, risk and protective factors, and suggest possible causes. After enumerating the extent of the problem and hypothesizing possible causal factors, researchers search for effective treatments. Studies shift from describing the problem to testing treatments or interventions. The ultimate goal is to develop an evidence-base of scientific knowledge to effectively treat, prevent, or eradicate the disease.

PUBLICATION BIAS

In reviewing past literature, the researcher must assess the quality of the research article. *Publication bias* is the tendency for journal editors to select certain types of studies over others for publication. Each professional journal has an impact factor, a number ranking that indicates how much the journal influences the field of interest. Impact factors are calculated by the total number of times articles are cited by researchers in a certain year divided by the total number of possible citations from the preceding years. Among medical journals in 2017, The *New England Journal of Medicine* scored an impact factor of 79.258, *The Lancet* scored 53.254, and the *Journal of the American Medical Association* scored 47.661. Higher scores indicate greater influence in the field of practice. To achieve desirable ranking, editors prefer groundbreaking studies, studies that will attract attention and are likely to yield high numbers of citations. This preference creates publication bias. Editors will gravitate toward studies with statistically significant results, studies by well-known researchers in the field, and studies supporting popular or novel ideas in the field. Publication bias can restrict published articles and limit knowledge of a topic.

With many, many submissions to choose from, editors are likely to reject studies of treatments and interventions that do not demonstrate statistical significance.

Knowing this, many researchers will not waste time writing reports of studies that did not prove their hypothesis. The lack of reporting is a problem. In the world of professional practice, it is important to know what does not work. For example, in the 1990s youth violence rates increased rapidly. Voters pressured politicians to implement programs to control youth violence. Boot camps were popular. Families and communities sent troubled youth to residential pseudo-military training camps. When researchers studied boot camps, they found the intervention did not work and could cause more harm than good. Boot camp staff modeled aggressive behavior teaching participants that violence was normal and acceptable. Boot camps did not work to reduce violence. With limited resources for mental health treatment and intervention, patients, families, and communities must make wise decisions regarding which programs to support. If researchers do not report studies of programs that do not work, the general public will continue to invest in these programs. Publication bias toward positive, statistically significant results creates a false impression and violates the idea of scientific research as the honest pursuit of knowledge. In reflecting on his own experiments, Thomas Edison said, "I have not failed. I have found 10,000 ways that won't work" (Elkhorne 1967). Failure, knowing what does not work, is just as important as knowing what does work.

The second type of publication bias, focusing on selected names in the field blocks other researchers from publishing and limits novel insights (see Matthew Effect and Matilda Effect in Chapter 8). When the same individuals are published repeatedly, knowledge becomes insular. Bias toward famous scholars also puts pressure on those who are trying to break through the ranks. This pressure can lead to scientific misconduct. William Summerlin and Eric Poehlman (Chapter 6) are examples of what happens when researchers feel pressured to "publish or perish."

The third type of bias, publishing studies promoting fashionable philosophy, has been called into question by a number of scholarly publishing sting operations. During the *science wars*, Alan Sokal, a physics professor at New York University performed a sting operation to call out publication bias in the social sciences. The science wars were intellectual debates between social scientists and natural scientists. Social scientists questioned the certainty of science in fields such as biology, chemistry, physics, and geology while natural scientists questioned the scientific merits of cultural studies. Editors of *Social Text*, a Duke University Press journal issued a call for articles on the science wars. Sokal wanted to show that *Social Text* editors were biased toward articles that forwarded postmodernist philosophy. He created a nonsensical article using all of the appropriate resources and terminology. The article, "Transgressing the Boundaries: Towards a Transformative Hermeneutics of Quantum Gravity" claimed that reality does not exist and is a "social and linguistic construct" (Sokal 1996, 217). The article was published in May and Sokal immediately announced that the article was a hoax. In their defense, the *Social Text* editors reported that Sokal's manuscript was poorly written and that he refused to make the requested edits. They published his article because it was the only one submitted by a natural scientist. Scholars stand divided on the Sokal Affair. Some say that Sokal acted unethically, violating scientific integrity by submitting a fabricated study. Others say that Sokal's submission revealed flaws in the academic publishing system. A number of subsequent publishing stings raise the same concerns and questions of how publication biases influence knowledge, further research, and practice.

STUDY 329

Publication bias encourages selective reporting. Study 329 is an extreme case of selective reporting with fatal consequences. Study 329 was a double blind, randomized controlled trial comparing the effectiveness of paroxetine (Paxil), imipramine (Tofranil), and a placebo in the treatment of clinical depression among teenagers. Paxil is a selective serotonin, reuptake inhibitor approved for use in 1992 and sold by GlaxoSmithKline (GSK). Imipramine is a tricyclic antidepressant developed in the 1950s and sold by Ciba-Geigy, now Novartis International AG. GSK funded Study 329 at 12 North American psychiatric centers. From April 1994 to March 1997, study personnel enrolled 275 adolescents, ages 12–18 years old into the eight-week study. All participants met the study criteria of major depression in the previous eight weeks. The acute phase of the study was followed by a six-month continuation period. The purpose of the continuation period was to determine safety of the drug with extended use and to estimate the relapse rates of depressive symptoms. From GSK's perspective, study results were not good. Paxil did not significantly reduce symptoms of depression. Nevertheless, GSK hired a ghostwriter, Sally K. Laden to write up the results for publication. Laden's manuscript concluded that Paxil demonstrated significant improvement in depressive symptom scores compared to the placebo and that imipramine was not significantly different from the placebo. Withdrawal rates due to adverse effects were 9.7 percent for Paxil, 6.9 percent for the placebo, and 31.5 percent for imipramine (Keller et al. 2001). Initially, the manuscript was rejected by the *Journal of the American Medical Association* and later accepted by the *Journal of the American Academy of Child and Adolescent Psychiatry*. GSK quickly sought and received approval to market Paxil for use in adolescents. Paxil quickly became the top-selling antidepressant in the nation with sales of $340 million (Restoring Invisible and Abandoned Trials Team n.d.).

Horrific cases of suicide by young people on Paxil or Paxil-similar substances started to emerge. Kara Jaye-Anne Otter took Paxil for eight months. Her parents felt pressured to put her on medication by school personnel. During Kara's Paxil regimen, her mother noticed increasing agitation. She requested psychiatric inpatient care and evaluation for another treatment regimen. Kara's psychiatrist dismissed the request. On June 7, 2001, the 12-year-old left a note for her parents and died by suicide. Other cases included Eric Harris who was on the SSRI Luvox at the time of the Columbine school attack and 18-year-old Sharise Gatchell. Gatchell started taking the UK equivalent of Paxil, Seroxat, 17 days before she died by suicide. As more news reports of young suicides emerged, grieving parents and doctors encouraged the British Medicines and Healthcare Products Regulatory Agency and the U.S. Food and Drug Administration (FDA) to launch investigations. The British group quickly banned the use of Paxil in children. The longer FDA investigation found:

- GSK promoted the use of Paxil to treat depression in youth under the age of 18 even though the drug had never been approved for pediatric use.

- GSK published an article that claimed Paxil effectively treated depression in patients under 18 years even though results did not show effectiveness (Study 329).

- GSK neglected to report or publicize two other studies that showed Paxil was ineffective.

- GSK sponsored dinners, lunch, and spa programs for potential prescribers in order to promote the use of Paxil in children.

GSK was also found guilty of withholding information on two other drugs and ordered to pay $1 billion in criminal fines and $2 million in civil settlements. The company was excused from admitting any wrongdoing. The *New York Times* reports Paxil sales at $11.6 billion during the period in question (Thomas and Schmidt 2012). In 2015, the RIAT (restoring invisible and abandoned trials) group sorted through volumes of Study 329 data. Reanalysis showed the misclassification of adverse events and no clear evidence of Paxil effectiveness. Five of the six adverse events labeled "emotional lability" were suicidal thinking or behavior (Le Noury et al. 2016). GSK stands by the original study results. GSK study authors dispute the RIAT review, and the *Journal of the American Academy of Child and Adolescent Psychiatry* refuses to retract the article. This type of selective reporting is a form of fraudulent science. In addition to the horrific clinical outcomes, selective reporting influences other research. Other researchers may have tried to replicate the study on effectiveness of Paxil and failed, wasting time and exposing study participants to unknown harm.

DUPLICATE PUBLISHING

Duplicate publishing, *redundant publishing*, or *self-plagiarism* is the repeat publication of a full article or portions of an article by the original author. When professional journals existed in hard copy only, redundant publication was acceptable. Publishing in multiple venues allowed the author to reach different professional groups. For example, an article on youth violence is of interest to public health professionals, sociologists, and criminal justice scholars. A study of programs to prevent youth violence may have been published in different journals to reach a wide variety of interested audiences. With easy access to research through online databases, duplicate publishing is now considered academic fraud (Scanlon 2007). Duplicate publishing has legal, ethical, and scientific implications. Since impact factor depends on number of citations, the journal loses citations and impact factor ranking when an article is published in multiple venues. Depending on the publisher, self-plagiarism could violate copyright law agreement. Journals invest a lot of time and resources reviewing submissions, sending manuscripts out for peer review, summarizing suggested edits, and following up with authors. With print journals, this process could take up to six months. Franz J. Ingelfinger, editor of *The New England Journal of Medicine*, expressed frustration with authors who went through the editing process with the journal and then used the editorial feedback to publish in other venues (Ingelfinger 1970). From his experiences in working with authors, Ingelfinger created a rule that no more than 10 percent of the text of an article should overlap with other publications or media releases. Scholarly journals apply the Ingelfinger Rule to ensure that their journal provides novel information. In scholarly publishing, once an author agrees to publish with a scholarly publisher, the publisher owns the copyright of the work. Publishing the article again is copyright infringement.

Duplicate publishing is unethical because it tricks readers, reviewers, and journalists into thinking that the scholar has done more research, published more articles, or enjoyed more citations than actually exist. From a scientific perspective, duplicate publishing crowds the field giving the appearance of multiple studies when in fact there was only one study. A review of 660 articles in three surgical journals found that one out of six articles represented some form of redundancy (Schein and Paladugu 2001). Three percent of the articles were word for word the same, and 7.6 percent were almost the same. The reviewers found high rates of *salami slicing*, where researchers take a large data set and break it down into separate sets in order to create several articles. The articles appear to be different studies, yet they are not. A red flag to duplicate publishing or salami slicing is if the author publishes hundreds or thousands of research articles. Good research takes time. If an article is identified as a redundant publication, the publisher may retract the article. Retraction means that the article is withdrawn and no longer available. To retract an article, the editor publishes a statement noting that the article should no longer be considered a valid source of scientific information. Future access to online copies of the article may be blocked. Journal editors do not like retractions. Retractions waste resources and effort and reflect poorly on the journal. Editors may blacklist an author with a retracted article. Retraction also reflects poorly on the researcher and coauthors. Other scientists are reluctant to cite the scholarly contributions of someone who has had an article retracted. The author and coauthors lose peer recognition.

Some scholars question whether self-plagiarism is possible. Plagiarism is defined as taking credit for the words or ideas of another author. With self-plagiarism, the author is not taking credit for someone else's work. The work is his or her own. Therefore, each case of self-plagiarism is decided separately, based on amount of overlap, intention, and whether the journal editors were aware of the redundancy. There are a few exceptions to the Ingelfinger Rule. Some journals republish landmark studies as a way to honor the anniversary of a speech, event, or discovery of historical significance. Editors also publish policy statements or practice guidelines to facilitate dissemination. This form of intentional copublication is acceptable practice.

MEGAJOURNALS AND PREDATORY PUBLISHERS

The internet created opportunities for individuals to disseminate research articles or other material through electronic venues. *Megajournals* are online publishers who aim for high outreach and a high number of publications through low selectivity of articles. *Predatory publishers* are low-quality, online publishers who charge authors to upload articles, conference presentations, or other material to their website for high fees. The groups are referred to as predatory publishers because they prey upon unsuspecting academics desperate to publish. Predatory publishers masquerade as legitimate scholarly publishing venues. However, article processing charges (APCs) are much higher than the actual cost of managing the operation. Fees are calculated by the journal, number of pages, and type of images. The unsuspecting researcher could pay from $250 to over $9,000 per article. Nine thousand dollars seems like a lot of money. However, some see it as an investment in acquiring tenure and promotion. Ten publications at $9,000 each ($90,000) is a small investment for a job that could pay approximately $4.8 million over a lifetime. A few predatory publishers offer an "all you can publish" option for an annual fee. Once an article is published online by a predatory publisher, the author holds the copyright. However, this does not mean the writer can use the work again in a legitimate press. Most scholarly journals will not accept an article for publication after it has already been published somewhere else. In some cases, researchers may pay for multiple articles in order to give the appearance of having more publications. *Predatory* is a misnomer for researchers who are attempting to game the system by publishing with predatory publishers. *Vanity publishing* is a more accurate term because the authors are intentionally paying to publish work that would probably not meet the selection criteria of legitimate scholarly press.

Charging a fee to publish online is not unusual. With the advent of online services, many large publishing houses now offer authors the opportunity to publish articles as open access. Open access means that readers who do not subscribe to the journal or who do not have access through library databases can view the article free of charge. Since publishers lose money by not charging the reader to access the article, the journal asks the author to cover the cost of publishing. Open access charges in a scholarly journal range from $150 to $4,000. Researchers may opt to pay the fee if they feel that their study offers new findings that will greatly advance the discipline and they want to disseminate their results to as wide an audience as possible. Submissions must still pass the peer review and editing process.

Predatory journals exist for the sole purpose of generating revenue. Peer review is often weak or nonexistent. If an author pays the fee, they can upload pretty much anything to the website. More than a few people have tested the criteria of predatory journals through satirical pranks. Professor of health policy at Curtin University, Australia, Dr. Mike Daube nominated his Staffordshire terrier Olivia "Ollie" Doll as editor with several predatory publishers. With research interests in the "benefits of abdominal massage for medium-sized canines" and "avian propinquity to canines in metropolitan suburbs," Ollie was successfully appointed to the editorial boards of seven medical journals (O'Leary 2017). In 2017, science blogger Neuroskeptic submitted the article "Mitochondria: Structure, Function and Clinical Relevance" to nine journals. The manuscript was submitted by Dr. Lucas McGeorge and Dr. Annette Kin. The paper plagiarized quotes from Star Wars and freely mixed and confused actual biological terms with fictional entities. For example, "Midi-chlorians are microscopic life-forms that reside in all living cells—without the midi-chlorians, life couldn't exist, and we'd have no knowledge of the force. Midichlorial disorders often erupt as brain diseases, such as autism" (Neuroskeptic 2017). Mitochondria are organelles that provide body cells with energy. Midi-chlorians are fictional microscopic life forms that give Jedi warriors their power to interface with the Force. Neuroskeptic took much of the text from Wikipedia, slightly rearranging the words and substituting terms. In the methods section, Neuroskeptic reported, "The majority of the text of this paper was Rogeted." Rogeted is the act of taking a published work and replacing some of the words with synonyms so that the text is not detected by an electronic plagiarism detector. Rogeting is a form of plagiarism because it takes the ideas and structure of the original author and presents the information as original work by the plagiarist. The Star Wars manuscript was accepted by four journals. One journal requested a $360 publication fee. (The author did not pay.) The other three journals published the article without fee, and Dr. Lucas McGeorge was invited to serve on the editorial board of one of the journals.

John H. McCool is founder and editor-in-chief of Precision Scientific Editing, a service assisting researchers to publish in high impact journals. McCool is on a mission to expose predatory publishing. His initial attempts in calling attention to the issues with predatory publishing were unsuccessful. He decided to take more extreme measures. In 2016, McCool received an email from *Urology & Nephrology Open Access Journal* seeking submissions. McCool is not a medical doctor or a urologist. Using the fictitious name of a doctor on the television show Seinfeld, McCool wrote a case study on "uromycitisis." Uromycitisis is a fictional disease, an excuse given by Seinfeld when he is caught urinating in public by a security guard. The paper was approved for publication with minor revisions for a fee of $799 plus tax. McCool did not pay the fee.

Predatory journals give the illusion of legitimacy. Inexperienced, gullible writers, eager to publish are vulnerable to unsolicited requests for submissions resulting in financial loss and loss of legitimate research. Predatory publishers rob young scientists of their time and talent. Years of effort on a research project may be lost because the scientist published in a questionable journal. For science, the lack of selectivity in publishing and poor peer review complicate the process of building a body of knowledge. Students and future researchers waste time reading, analyzing, or attempting to replicate studies without scientific merit.

CHERRY-PICKING THE LITERATURE

Cherry-picking is the selective use of information or facts. In terms of the literature review, cherry-picking occurs when the scientist overlooks some published research or facts in order to select literature that supports personal or professional philosophy. Cherry-picking the literature is slightly different from pathological science. Pathological science is the manipulation of study results. Cherry-picking is bias in collecting or reviewing existing sources of information. The selective use of materials may be unintentional or intentional.

Unintentional bias may result from a limited review, where the writer relies heavily on only a few sources. One way to avoid unintentional bias is to expand the literature review to a greater number and variety of resources. At the very minimum, the literature review should contain 10–12 quality scholarly resources. The type of resource can also create bias. Heavy reliance on internet sites creates bias because internet sources are not always accurate. Content is even less accurate when the website is selling a product. If the reviewer prefers to rely mainly on internet sources, it is best to use .org, .gov, or .edu websites and to avoid commercial websites. The strongest, most accurate literature reviews include a variety of traditional resources, such as journal articles and up-to-date textbooks, and reputable online resources, such as professional or government organizations.

Intentional biases are often the result of political or personal opinions. The researcher may dismiss some literature or argue strongly against it in order to support the desired belief. Regardless of intentionality, biases can result in incomplete evidence, misguided research studies, and further misinformation shared with other researchers. To avoid bias, the literature review should contain a good mix of scholarly references, original studies in peer-reviewed journals, and reference books, and the author should present the information in a fair, impartial way.

Curing Homosexuality

Conversion therapy, attempting to change someone's sexual orientation is an example of how religion and politics bias health research and patient treatment. Social stigmas against sexual minorities originated in the Middle Ages of Western civilization when the church condemned non-procreative sexual activities as unnatural and immoral. Prostitution, masturbation, sexual acts between unmarried couples, homosexuality, and heterosexual intercourse with the female on top were considered sins. As secular institutions replaced the church as the primary social authority, laws were developed that mimicked the social attitudes of the time. Homosexuality became illegal in many countries. Interestingly, laws tended to overlook females and focus on male homosexuality. The development of medicine and psychology as professional disciplines brought slightly more accepting attitudes. While many leading psychologists viewed homosexuality as perversion, Freud was known to have consoled a mother who was worried about her son's sexual orientation. Freud noted that throughout history homosexuals contributed greatly to society.

The first version of the American Psychological Association's *Diagnostic and Statistical Manual* (*DSM-I*) listed homosexuality as a "sociopathic personality disturbance." In the 1960s and 1970s, psychologists Irving Bieber and Charles Socarides forwarded the idea that homosexuality could be cured. In an article in the *Journal of Consulting and Clinical Psychology*, Bieber wrote, "As to the assumption that homosexuality is normal: Over the many years of my work with many colleagues on this subject, we have found no supporting evidence. . . . I shall not offer a critique of her [Evelyn Hooker] studies; others have already done so. I shall, instead, refer to my own work" (Bieber 1976, 163). The psychoanalyst dismissed the work of others and recommended conversion or reparative therapy. Based on this theory, efforts to change sexual orientation emerged, such as prayer, bible study, individual or group therapy, surgery, aversion therapy, excessive exercise, and electroshock therapy. In 1977, researchers from the University of Georgia identified 37 studies evaluating sexual orientation change efforts (SOCE) for scientific merit and effectiveness (Adams and Sturgis 1977). One study of aversion therapy induced nausea by injecting male participants with emetine, apomorphone, and caffeine-apomorphone combinations and then showed them pictures of naked men. At a subsequent visit, the participants were injected with testosterone to increase sexual drive and shown pictures of naked women. Of the original 67 participants, 20 refused to complete the study. A later review of SOCE studies performed between 1960 and 2007 concluded that most of the 55 studies contained major methodological flaws (American Psychological Association 2009). Common flaws involved dependence on self-report of sexual orientation as an outcome or inclusion of participants from religious groups that openly advocated for conversion therapy. Reviewers believe that the study participants may have felt pressured to report what the researchers wanted them to report or were embarrassed to acknowledge ongoing homosexual desires.

By the 1970s, civil rights activists questioned the classification of homosexuality as a disorder and criticized psychiatry and medicine for pathologizing healthy human behavior. Activists cited the medical disorder of drapetomania as an example of overreach. Identified in 1851 by Dr. Samuel A. Cartwright, drapetomania was considered a mental disorder of African slaves. The disorder caused slaves to escape captivity or attempt to escape by running away. Cartwright recommended the medical treatment of severe beating with a whip or removal of the large toes. Long after the Emancipation Proclamation, drapetomania appeared in medical texts. The example allowed psychologists to see how personal biases influenced knowledge. LGBT rights activists Frank Kameny, Barbara Gittings, and John Fryer were instrumental in shifting American Psychological Association (APA) members' attitudes and understanding of homosexuality. The advocates offered workshop sessions at APA conferences and explained the consequences of labeling same-gender sexual orientation as a psychiatric illness. In 1973, APA's Board of Trustees voted to remove homosexuality from the DSM. The decision was confirmed by APA member vote. Despite the declassification and depathologization, SOCE continue to be offered. Several studies with small populations suggest that experiences with SOCE and interaction with SOCE practitioners may lower self-esteem and increase feelings of social rejection resulting in depression, suicide attempt, or difficulties with intimacy (Shidlo and Schroeder 2002). Bieber's quote shows how his work and ideas were insular. He had few qualms in declaring the outright rejection of other research and although his work and ideas were discredited, the vilification of homosexuality continues to harm the mental health of LGBTQ people. Selective use of the literature, cherry-picking, can have implications beyond the research.

Scientists depend on other scientists to provide accurate information. The literature review establishes a provenance of ideas for future exploration. To create the literature review, the scientist performs an extensive search of the literature, reads, organizes, and conveys the information to the reader, and builds connections between past research and the proposed project. The author must be very careful to ensure that only scholarly and reputable sources are used because the review forms the foundation for a project. Neglecting to perform a literature review or skipping over the literature review leads to poorly devised studies and possible scientific misconduct. Additionally, hoaxing, forging, pathological science, fraud, duplicate publishing, and vanity publishing can mislead other scientists into doing studies that are not warranted or are potentially harmful to patients and study participants. Writing a strong literature review is one of the most important parts of a research study.

FURTHER READING

Adams, Henry E., and Ellie T. Sturgis. 1977. "Status of Behavioral Reorientation Techniques in the Modification of Homosexuality: A Review." *Psychological Bulletin* 84 (6): 1171–88.

American Psychological Association, Task Force on Appropriate Therapeutic Responses to Sexual Orientation. 2009. "Report of the American Psychological Association Task Force on Appropriate Therapeutic Responses to Sexual Orientation." Accessed August 25, 2018. https://www.apa.org/pi/lgbt/resources/therapeutic-response.pdf

Bérubé, Michael, and Alan Sokal. 2000. "The Sokal Hoax." In *The Sokal Hoax: The Sham That Shook the Academy*, edited by Lingua Franca, 139–47. Lincoln: University of Nebraska Press.

Bieber, I. 1976. "A Discussion of 'Homosexuality: The Ethical Challenge.'" *Journal of Consulting and Clinical Psychology* 44 (2): 163–66.

Bohannon, John. 2014. "Study of Massive Preprint Archive Hints at the Geography of Plagiarism." *Science.* Accessed August 21, 2018. https://www.sciencemag.org/news/2014/12/study-massive-preprint-archive-hints-geography-plagiarism

Citron, Daniel T., and Paul Ginsparg. 2015. "Patterns of Text Reuse in a Scientific Corpus." *Proceedings of the National Academy of Sciences of the United States of America* 112 (1): 25–30.

Drescher, Jack. 2015. "Out of DSM: Depathologizing Homosexuality." *Behavioral Sciences* 5 (4): 565–75.

Elkhorne, J. L. 1967. "Edison: The Fabulous Drone." *73 Magazine* XLVI (3) (March): 52–54.

Ford, Jeffry G. 2001. "Healing Homosexuals: A Psychologist's Journey through the Ex-gay Movement and the Pseudo-science of Reparative Therapy." *Journal of Gay & Lesbian Psychotherapy* 5 (3–4): 69–86.

"Influence of Sex on Heart-Disease." 1872. *The British Medical Journal* 1 (587): 347–347.

Ingelfinger, Franz J. 1970. "Medical Literature: The Campus without Tumult." *Science* 169 (3948): 831–37.

"Is Recycling Your Own Work Plagiarism?" Accessed August 14, 2019. https://www.turnitin.com/blog/is-recycling-your-own-work-plagiarism?utm_source=chronicle&utm_medium=email&utm_campaign=nov_campaign

Kantor, Martin. 2015. *Why a Gay Person Can't Be Made Un-gay: The Truth about Reparative Therapies*. Santa Barbara, CA: Praeger.

Keller, Martin B., Neal D. Ryan, Michael Strober, Rachel G. Klein, Stan P. Kutcher, Boris Birmaher, Owen R. Hagino, et al. 2001. "Efficacy of Paroxetine in the Treatment of Adolescent Major Depression: A Randomized, Controlled Trial." *Journal of the American Academy of Child & Adolescent Psychiatry* 40 (7): 762–72.

Le Noury, Joanna, John M. Nardo, David Healy, Jon Jureidini, Melissa Raven, Catalin Tufanaru, and Elia Abi-Jaoude. 2016. "Study 329 Continuation Phase: Safety and Efficacy of Paroxetine and Imipramine in Extended Treatment of Adolescent Major Depression." *International Journal of Risk & Safety in Medicine* 28 (3): 143–61.

Lifton, Robert Jay. 1986. *The Nazi Doctors: Medical Killing and the Psychology of Genocide*. New York: Basic Books.

McConaghy, N., and R. F. Barr. 1973. "Classical, Avoidance and Backward Conditioning Treatments of Homosexuality." *British Journal of Psychiatry* 122 (567) (February): 151–62.

McCool, John H. 2017. "Why I Published in a Predatory Journal: Our Totally Bogus Case Report Swiftly Passed Muster, with Only Minor Revisions Requested." *Scientist* 31 (6): 23.

Neuroskeptic. 2017. "Predatory Journals Hit by 'Star Wars' Sting." *Discover*, July 22. Accessed May 5, 2018. http://blogs.discovermagazine.com /neuroskeptic/2017/07/22/predatory-journals-star-wars-sting /#.XROFrsQpBPZ

O'Leary, Cathy. 2017. "Is This the World's Smartest Canine? Or Has Science Gone to the Dogs?" *The Western Australian*, May 21. Accessed April 27, 2018. https://thewest.com.au/news/health/is-this-the-worlds-smartest -canine-or-has-science-gone-to-the-dogs-ng-b88479075z

OR Manager. 2007. "OR Logistics: Learning from FedEx." *OR Manager* 23 (11) (November 1): 12–13.

Pearce, R. M. 1912. "Chance and the Prepared Mind." *Science* 35 (912): 941–56.

Restoring Invisible and Abandoned Trials Team. n.d. "Restoring Study 329." Accessed January 24, 2019. https://study329.org/

Scanlon, Patrick M. 2007. "Song from Myself: An Anatomy of Self Plagiarism." *Plagiary* (January): 57–66.

Schein, Moshe, and Ramesh Paladugu. 2001. "Redundant Surgical Publications: Tip of the Iceberg?" *Surgery* 129 (6): 655–61.

Shidlo, Ariel, and Michael Schroeder. 2002. "Changing Sexual Orientation: A Consumers' Report." *Professional Psychology: Research and Practice* 33 (3): 249–59.

Sokal, Alan D. 1996. "Transgressing the Boundaries: Toward a Transformative Hermeneutics of Quantum Gravity." *Social Text* 46/47: 217–52.

Thomas, Katie, and Michael S. Schmidt. 2012. "Glaxo Agrees to Pay $3 Billion in Fraud Settlement." Accessed August 25, 2018. https://www.nytimes .com/2012/07/03/business/glaxosmithkline-agrees-to-pay-3-billion-in -fraud-settlement.html

U.S. Department of Justice. 2012. "GlaxoSmithKline to Plead Guilty and Pay $3 Billion to Resolve Fraud Allegations and Failure to Report Safety Data." *Justice News*, July 2. Accessed August 18, 2019. https://www.justice.gov /opa/pr/glaxosmithkline-plead-guilty-and-pay-3-billion-resolve-fraud -allegations-and-failure-report

Weinblatt, Eve, Sam Shapiro, and Charles W. Frank. 1973. "Prognosis of Women with Newly Diagnosed Coronary Heart Disease—A Comparison with Course of Disease among Men." *American Journal of Public Health* 63 (7) (July 1973): 577–93.

The Writing Center, University of North Carolina at Chapel Hill. n.d. "Literature Reviews." Accessed June 1, 2018. https://writingcenter.unc.edu/tips-and -tools/literature-reviews/

FOUR

Study Design

The research design is the blueprint of the scientific study. Much like the architect's blueprint, the design defines the overall concept of the project. The terms *study design* and *study methods* are related but refer to distinctly different aspects of the study. Study design is the plan for the experiment. Study methods are the step-by-step procedures. For example, *ethnography* is a type of qualitative study design that investigates the culture of a particular group or subgroup of people. Examples of ethnographic studies might be exploring the camaraderie of firefighters, social support of isolated communities in rural Appalachia, or experiences in transitioning from medical student to qualified doctor. Study methods describe how the researcher collected the data—the who, what, where, when, and how of the study. Study methods are written as instructions for other scientists, students, and readers to understand how a study was conducted. For example, "the primary investigator, a graduate student in public health, interviewed 20 adolescents between the ages of 16 and 18 on attitudes toward vaping. The interviews were held in a designated private area of the local community center and lasted approximately 45–60 minutes. Interviews were conducted between June 15, 2019, and August 15, 2019." Study methods are distinctive to each study. There are many different ways to study a particular topic of interest. The final determination of design depends on the purpose of the study, research hypothesis, available resources, timeline for completion, suggested next steps from the literature review, and the most logical approach to the issue. There is no perfect study design. Every study design has advantages and limitations. Developing the study design is one of the most creative steps of the scientific method.

INDUCTIVE, DEDUCTIVE, AND ABDUCTIVE REASONING

To determine the appropriate study design, the researcher considers the purpose of the study and how to collect evidence that will lead to a logical conclusion. The study conclusion must be based on rational interpretation of the results and what they mean within the larger context of what is already known. This process occurs through three types of reasoning. Scientists primarily use inductive and deductive reasoning. Inductive reasoning examines individual cases in order to draw general conclusions. An example of inductive reasoning is Dr. Sigmund Freud's research into psychic structure. Freud developed psychoanalytic theory based on his interactions with individual patients. He initially observed and published case studies of patients in *Studies on Hysteria* (1895) and *The Interpretation of Dreams* (1900). Deductive reasoning starts with an overall premise or theory and tests the theory in individual cases. In his later work, Freud used deductive reasoning, starting with the theory and applying the theory to individual cases. Freud applied his earlier observations to the larger population of people with and without mental illness. He published deductive application in *The Psychopathology of Everyday Life* (1901) and *Three Essays on the Theory of Sexuality* (1905). Using both inductive and deductive reasoning, Freud provided groundbreaking insights into the human psyche.

Inductive studies are exploratory, examining single or small groups of individuals in order to discover shared characteristics. Study results are reported as detailed descriptions highlighting common themes or experiences of study participants who have directly or indirectly experienced the phenomenon of interest. The disadvantage of inductive research is that it makes assumptions that may be skewed. In Freud's case, his ideas were based on a clinical population, people with mental illness at the turn of the twentieth century. The experiences, lifestyle, and culture of Freud's patients were unique and do not apply to all people of that era. Whereas inductive research may be viewed as a bottom-up approach, deductive research is a top-down approach. Deductive research starts with a general idea and applies the idea on an individual basis. An example of deductive research is taking Freud's ideas on the psychosexual stages of development and testing his theory in a sample of children.

A third form of reasoning, abductive reasoning draws connections between partial observations in order to develop the most likely explanation. Abductive reasoning is a common method of everyday problem-solving. This type of logic is used when the individual does not have all of the information needed to make a definitive decision yet must make a decision. Abductive reasoning examines the evidence collected by a particular investigation and draws the most logical conclusion based on the results. An example of abductive reasoning is jury cases. The jurors are only given the evidence presented in the courtroom. They may not have all of the information that they need to determine guilt or innocence, yet they still must decide. While each form of logic is useful, the typical progression of research is to study individual cases (inductive), develop theory, and then test the theory as a research hypothesis in a larger group (deductive).

In addition to using inductive and deductive reasoning to draw logical conclusions, scientists use inductive and deductive reasoning to design the research study. Deductive experiments, commonly referred to as empirical research, test a research hypothesis. The *research hypothesis* is a specific, clear, and testable statement of what ought to be observed as an outcome of the experiment. Empirical studies test the hypothesis by measuring, counting and comparing the variable of interest in the experimental group to either another point in time (pre-intervention) or another group of participants (control group). In order to test the hypothesis, deductive studies must use samples that are large enough to show statistical significance. A small sample or a small difference between samples may not be enough to show a difference and therefore to prove or disprove the hypothesis. Inductive studies are qualitative. Qualitative studies seek to answer a research question in order to gain deeper insight and understanding of an issue. Small populations are used in qualitative studies so that the researcher can delve into the issue. Qualitative studies do not test a research hypothesis. Qualitative results develop a research hypothesis for future study. In summary, deductive or empirical studies tend to be quantitative or number based, while inductive studies tend to be qualitative or focused on detailed themes or descriptions. The majority of studies are either inductive (qualitative) or deductive (quantitative). Studies that are both inductive and deductive are known as *mixed methods* studies.

PROVING CAUSALITY

Identifying the cause of a disease or public health problem is a major step toward preventing future cases. Therefore, a lot of medical research focuses on finding the causes of a particular disease. The classic example of proving causality is Sir Austin Bradford Hill and Sir William Shaboe Richard Doll's discovery of cigarette smoking as the major cause of lung cancer. Prior to Hill and Doll's research, cigarettes were marketed as health enhancing. New York Yankees baseball player Mickey Mantle advertised Viceroy cigarettes. Six-time Major League Baseball All Star Jackie Robinson appeared in ads for Chesterfield cigarettes. Lucky Strike cigarettes claimed that 20,679 doctors recommended Luckies to protect against cough. Cigarette manufacturers claimed that smoking eased breathing, protected the throat, and helped the smoker maintain healthy weight. As the rates of lung cancer increased, medical doctors raised concerns about the link to smoking. Tobacco companies responded by dismissing the concerns or attacking the doctors. In 1954, Hill and Doll published their landmark study, "The Mortality of Doctors in Relation to Their Smoking Habits." The study followed 40,564 doctors over approximately two and a half years. Of the doctors who died of lung cancer, all were smokers, and the more one smoked, the greater the risk of lung cancer. The Hill and Doll study is a landmark study because the researchers followed a highly reliable, healthy population over time. Doctors are considered a reliable source of health information, well qualified to report health risks and exposures. Tracking the doctors' health over time meant that the researchers could rule out other possible causes. Once study results were published, other researchers quickly replicated and confirmed the relationship between cigarette smoking and lung cancer. In 1964, the surgeon general issued the *Report on Smoking and Health*. The report called for a health warning on all cigarette packages and banned cigarette advertising in broadcast media. Identifying a major cause of lung cancer allowed health professionals to plan smoking cessation and smoking prevention programs and counter the increasing rates of respiratory disease.

A common logical fallacy in reporting research results is the misconception that correlation implies causation. Correlation is a statistical calculation that enumerates the direction and strength of the relationship between two variables. In a survey asking participants about history of smoking and lung cancer, the Pearson's correlation (r) was +0.716. This result means that smoking is moderately (0.7 is a moderate correlation; the closer r is to 1.0, the stronger the relationship) and positively (0.7 is positive, not negative) associated with lung cancer. Because the survey looked at both variables at the same point in time, the statistician cannot say that lung cancer causes smoking or smoking causes lung cancer, only that the two variables are positively or directly related. As one variable goes up, the other variable goes up, or as one variable goes down, the other variable goes down. If the variables were negatively or indirectly related, one variable would decrease as the other variable increases. With significant correlations, the simple (and hasty) assumption is that one variable causes the other. However, this is flawed logic. Large data sets often reveal significant correlations where there is no actual relationship. Tyler Vigen (2015) made a sport out of scanning large data sets to find funny and meaningless correlations. Vigen found an almost perfect correlation (r = 0.99789126) between U.S. spending on science, space, and technology and suicides by hanging, strangulation, and suffocation. The relationship between number of people who drowned by falling into a pool directly correlates with the number of films actor Nicolas Cage appeared in (r = 0.666004). The number of letters in the winning word of Scripps National Spelling Bee correlates with the number of people killed by venomous spiders (r = 0.8057). Correlations suggest that two variables are related. They do not prove causality. Retrospective studies, studies that look backward in time, and correlational studies, studies that look at two variables at the same time, cannot demonstrate causality. Prospective studies, studies that follow participants over a period of time and collect data throughout that period, are the strongest study design in proving causality. This is why Hill and Doll's study of doctors was so important. The researchers monitored the doctors over time.

In 1965, Sir Bradford Hill proposed nine criteria for epidemiologists to determine if an observed association can be considered a causal relationship. The Bradford Hill criteria are:

1. *Strength of association:* The relationship between the causal factor and the outcome is statistically significant.

2. *Consistency:* The results are not an anomaly. Other scientists are able to reproduce the original study results.

3. *Specificity:* The relationship between cause and effect is distinct. The outcome cannot be explained by a third factor (i.e., the doctors did not consistently report another exposure that could account for increased rates of cancer).

4. *Temporality:* The causal factor occurs before the outcome (i.e., smoking comes before lung cancer).

5. *Biological gradient:* A dose response relationship exists where the greater the dose or exposure to the causal factor, the greater the outcome (i.e., the more cigarettes one smokes, the greater the risk of lung cancer).

6. *Plausibility:* The relationship makes sense with respect to the current body of knowledge on the mechanism of disease (i.e., it makes sense that inhaling strong chemicals would harm cilia lining the respiratory tract, irritate respiratory tissue, and trigger dysfunctional lung cell growth).

7. *Coherence:* Similar to biological plausibility, the causal relationship matches current information regarding what is known about diseases in general (i.e., tobacco smoke contains many toxic chemicals; toxins are known to cause a variety of human and animal diseases as well as fatality).

8. *Experiment:* Disease risk declines following cessation of exposure, planned treatment, or intervention (i.e., people who stop smoking can reduce their risk of lung cancer).

9. *Analogy:* A similar agent to the causal factor also results in the same outcome or a related outcome (i.e., exposure to asbestos also causes lung cancer).

The Hill and Doll study supported strength of association, temporality, specificity, and biological gradient. Other studies by independent researchers were required to support consistency, coherence, experiment, and analogy. In reviewing the conditions of causality, it becomes apparent that one study alone cannot prove causality. Proving causality requires multiple studies with different study designs.

The Antivaccination Campaign

The assumption of causality can have drastic effects. In 1998, doctors at the Royal Free Hospital and School of Medicine in London published a report of

12 children who presented with loss of previously acquired developmental skills (autism), diarrhea, and abdominal pain. The report appeared in the prestigious British medical journal, *The Lancet*. The authors found, "Onset of behavioral symptoms was associated by the parents, with measles, mumps, and rubella vaccination in eight of the 12 children" (Wakefield et al. 1998, 637). *The Lancet* article and a subsequent paper received little attention until one of the authors, Andrew Wakefield, appeared in a televised press conference featuring gastrointestinal research. Wakefield questioned whether the MMR vaccine was associated with autism. Journalists immediately jumped on the story. While scientists and health professionals debated Wakefield's science, some parents became reluctant to have their child immunized. In the United Kingdom, vaccination rates dropped and measles cases increased from 56 in 1998 to 1,370 in 2008 (Public Health England 2014). Several children died from complications due to measles. Many children were hospitalized.

Scientists around the world tried to test Wakefield's theory without success. By 2004, the scientific community concluded that there is no link between the MMR vaccine and autism. In 2006, the *Sunday Times* reported that Wakefield had earned more than $670,000 in consulting fees from attorneys representing parents who believed their children were harmed by the MMR vaccine. Wakefield's consultancy began prior to the 1998 publication. The U.K. General Medical Council revoked Wakefield's license due to ethical concerns. He was cleared of charges of professional misconduct for failing to disclose the conflict of interest to journal editors. Although 11 of the 12 coauthors issued a formal retraction of the article, the internet, news media, talk shows, and other popular sources continued to feature the story. Wakefield's antivaccination campaign is particularly strong among young parents who never witnessed the horrors of smallpox, typhoid, mumps, polio, and other vaccine preventable diseases. In the United States, one in five parents believe that vaccines cause autism (Freed et al. 2010). *New York Times* journalist Susan Dominus describes the former captain of his medical school's rugby team and head boy at an elite private school as, "One of the most reviled doctors of his generation, blamed directly or indirectly, depending on the accuser, for irresponsibly starting a panic of tragic repercussions: vaccination rates so low that childhood diseases once all but eradicated here—whooping cough and measles, among them—have re-emerged, endangering young lives" (Dominus 2011, 36). Wakefield assumed that autism and vaccinations were related because they occur around the same developmental period. His theory was based on the clinical observations of 12 children who were intentionally brought to the gastroenterology clinic and parents who wanted some explanation of why their child had stopped developing normally. In announcing his idea to the press, Wakefield violated the conditions of causality and bypassed scientific safeguards.

TYPES OF STUDY DESIGNS

Study designs may be confusing because there are multiple ways to classify designs (i.e., inductive, deductive, quantitative, qualitative, prospective, or retrospective). The key to understanding study design is to recognize the main categories of designs. Knowing the categories and the advantages and disadvantages of each category allows the researcher to determine the best design for a particular study. The main categories of research design are (a) qualitative field research (inductive), (b) descriptive or epidemiological, (c) true experimental (deductive), (d) quasi-experimental (deductive), and (e) evaluation design (inductive or deductive). Within each category are specific designs. Some designs only fit into one category. For example, ethnography is a qualitative design while pretest, posttest control group design is a true experimental design. Other designs fit into multiple categories depending on what data the researcher collects. *Survey research* may be true experimental, quasi-experimental, or qualitative.

There is an assumption among some natural scientists that true experimental studies are the gold standard of research. The assertion is that true experimental studies exhibit less bias in data collection and reporting than qualitative research. The Sokal Hoax was based on this bias (see chapter 3). In reality, each type of study design has advantages, limitations, and biases. Each study design offers a unique perspective on the topic of interest while adding to the current body of knowledge. The logical order of exploring an issue is to use a qualitative design to explore and define the issue followed by quantitative designs to measure the extent or impact of the problem and then an evaluation design to discover evidence-based treatment or prevention. In large studies, researchers may combine study designs.

Qualitative Studies

Qualitative studies may be used to describe emerging or re-emerging problems. These types of studies investigate an issue in-depth in order to acquire meaningful understanding. To collect data, the researcher goes to areas where the problem exists and interviews those affected by the issue. The practice of going into a community to collect data is referred to as *field research* because the researcher works in the field as opposed to a laboratory. Field research studies are carried out in much the same way as an investigative journalist. Field research may be quantitative, qualitative, or mixed methods. In qualitative research, field research is a dominant characteristic. Some of the major types of qualitative research are ethnography, phenomenology, hermeneutics, and interpretivism. Qualitative studies can be very personal, investigating behaviors that are difficult to measure through survey or other means.

The Tearoom Trade Study

In 1968, Robert Allan "Laud" Humphreys set out to deconstruct the stigma surrounding the sexual behavior of men who have sex with men (MSM). The Washington University in St. Louis student suspected that many of the men who engaged in homosexual encounters in public places lived a double life with heterosexual relationships. Given public stigma against homosexuality, Humphreys knew that he could not simply interview the men. He designed an ethnographic study where he offered to act as a lookout for men seeking impersonal sex in the restrooms of public parks, known as tearooms. Tearoom is slang for toilet room, t-room. The "Study of the Sociology of the Organization and Structure of Sexually Deviant Behavior in Public Restrooms" provided insight into the various hand signals and body language the men used to communicate to one another. Study results contradicted popular concerns that MSM prey on children or unsuspecting heterosexual men. The study provided better insight into this private behavior than if Humphreys had used a survey. The Tearoom Trade Study is best known for the second part of the study. While assuming the role of the "watch queen," Humphreys recorded the men's license plate numbers. A year later, he altered his identity, tracked the men to their home address, and visited the men in their homes posing as a social researcher. He collected data on age, marital status, and other social demographics. The second set of data was quantitative and used to show that many MSM live public lives as heterosexuals. The study is criticized for human participant protections. Humphreys failed to gain informed consent and failed to disclose the true nature of the study to the participants. Faculty at Washington University in St. Louis disputed the ethics of the research. Humphreys argued that the behavior occurred in a public place and therefore did not require informed consent. Some faculty resigned in protest. The Tearoom Trade Study is a famous study investigating a private, personal behavior that would have been difficult to study through other designs.

True Experimental and Quasi-Experimental Design

True experimental and quasi-experimental studies are used to test the effects of an experimental stimulus, also known as the independent variable (IV), on a dependent variable (DV). The independent variable could be a drug, treatment, or intervention. The dependent variable may be a trait, such as blood pressure, health behavior, or level of anxiety. True experimental and quasi-experimental studies tend to be quantitative or deductive. The researcher tests a hypothesis stating that as the independent variable is adjusted, the dependent variable will also vary. The main difference between true experimental and quasi-experimental is that true experimental studies have random assignment. Study participants or study samples are randomly assigned to the experimental or control group. The experimental group is the group that receives the stimulus whereas the control group does not receive the stimulus. Random assignment typically ensures that the groups are similar at baseline on whatever trait the researchers are comparing. Quasi-experimental studies are used when random assignment is not possible. With quasi-experimental studies, the researcher may only use one group and compare the dependent variable levels before and after the stimulus. For example, in the case where researchers are assessing the impact of a new playground on children's activity levels, it would be objectionable to randomly assign which children could play on the playground (experimental group) and which children could not play on the playground (control group). Comparing activity levels before and after the program supports the bioethical principle of justice. In some quasi-experimental studies, the researchers may use a comparison group (i.e., same age children from a neighborhood outside of the new playground's catchment area). With quasi-experimental studies, the researchers know that the groups may not be similar at baseline. The researcher may need to adjust the results statistically in order to minimize baseline differences. In the example of the playground, young females tend to be less active than males of the same age. If the groups vary greatly by gender, the researcher may have to adjust for differences in gender between the groups. The main advantage of true experimental and quasi-experimental studies is replicability. Replicability is the ability to replicate or repeat an experiment and get the same or similar results as the original study. Replicability is one of the conditions of causality. Replicability is high with true experimental and quasi-experimental studies because application of the IV and measurement of the DV occur under controlled conditions. The researcher carefully defines when and how the intervention or drug will be administered (the IV) and when and how data are collected (the DV). Under controlled conditions, the researcher is able to isolate the treatment and control groups from any variables that may influence the outcome. The ability to replicate a study supports the hypothesis and refutes the idea that the results occurred by chance. Disadvantages of true experimental and quasi-experimental studies are that the studies occur under controlled conditions. In real life conditions, external factors may influence the relationship between the DV and the IV. By controlling external factors, the researcher may not gain an accurate impression of the relationship.

As with other steps to the scientific method, there is the opportunity for scientists to manipulate true experimental or quasi-experimental experiments to prove a particular point. For example, the Comparison of Atypicals in First Episode study (described in chapter 2) compared newer antipsychotic medications. The study did not include older medications because there was no financial benefit to the pharmaceutical company if the study results proved that the older drugs were more effective than the newer drugs.

Georgia Pacific's Study of Asbestos Exposure

Manipulation of study design is a common ploy of businesses attempting to market products. In 1924, Dr. W. E. Cooke, pathologist at Wigan Infirmary, England, reported the case of a 33-year-old woman who died of severe lung fibrosis. The woman had worked in asbestos factories since the age of 13 (Cooke 1924). Her case was not unusual. Local doctors treated many long-term factory workers for lung disorders. They suspected that asbestos caused the lung problems. Asbestos is a group of fibrous minerals. The material is soft and pliable and does not corrode over time, making it great for insulating walls or pipes. Cooke's patient had extensive fibrosis of the lungs with noticeable hollow cavities. He also observed sharp pieces of mineral matter in the lungs. Cooke suggested that small fibers of asbestos could break off as dust and enter the body through the lungs. Over the next several decades, researchers investigated asbestos as an occupational health issue. One large-scale survey of 1,074 pipe coverers in U.S. Navy shipyards identified low rates of asbestosis, 0.29 percent (Fleischer et al. 1946). However, the study was limited by the fact that the shipyard had high employee turnover. Few study participants experienced long-term exposure.

In 1947, the American Conference of Governmental Industrial Hygienists recommended limiting exposure to asbestos. By 1955, Sir Richard Doll proved statistically that asbestos exposure caused lung cancer. In the United States, the leading medical researcher in asbestos-related diseases was Mount Sinai Hospital physician Irving J. Selikoff. Selikoff started his medical practice in Paterson, New Jersey. When the Asbestos Workers Union asked Selikoff to add their members to his clients, Selikoff noticed numerous cases of the lung disease mesothelioma. Selikoff conducted research on lung diseases, published numerous articles, and became very vocal about the dangers of asbestos. He quickly became the target of a smear campaign by the asbestos industry. The industry questioned his medical credentials and accused him of being biased and exaggerating the health effects of asbestos. It is now known that asbestos dust can be inhaled or ingested. Long-term exposure for 20–30 years can cause mesothelioma, lung cancer, laryngeal cancer, ovarian cancer, and other forms of cancer.

After World War II, demand for new, inexpensive homes created a construction boom. Population movement to once rural areas created demand for new schools, businesses, and other building projects. Bestwall Gypsum was one of several companies that manufactured drywall, plaster, and joint compounds. These products contained a type of asbestos known as chrysotile asbestos. In 1965, paper company Georgia-Pacific LLC (G-P) purchased Bestwall. G-P continued manufacturing products with asbestos even though asbestos was widely recognized as an occupational health hazard. Clarence Borel worked as an insulator from 1936 to 1969. He and coworkers questioned the safety of the heavy dust that layered their clothing, faces, and hands day after day. However, they were never given any safety instructions, and they assumed the dust was broken down within their bodies. Employees could request a respirator if they wanted one. However, the respirators were hot and uncomfortable, not conducive to working in Texas. Borel was diagnosed with asbestosis. In 1973, he successfully sued a group of manufacturers for breach of duty, failing to inform workers of the hazards associated with asbestos. He died of mesothelioma before the final court verdict. Over 60,000 workers followed suit (Morris 2013).

With potentially $1 billion of lawsuits at stake, G-P created a plan to cast doubt on the medical claims supporting the lawsuits. G-P paid $6 million to 18 scientists to publish studies refuting the hazards of asbestos. Thirteen studies financed by G-P were published between 2008 and 2012. It is not unusual for businesses to fund research into product development. This research was purposely flawed. G-P's director of toxicology and chemical management, Stewart E. Holm played a critical role in study development and reporting. The studies focused on short-term effects of exposure rather than long-term effects. The first study compared how long chrysotile asbestos fibers stayed in the body of laboratory rats (Bernstein et al. 2008). The study concluded that the lungs of rats exposed to chrysotile asbestos for six hours per day over five days did not differ from the lungs of control rats using filtered air. In 2010, G-P's researchers compared the short-term effects of chrysotile asbestos to amosite asbestos and concluded, "This study provides support that the sanded joint compound would not initiate an inflammatory response in the lung following inhalation and the chrysotile fibers present do not migrate to the pleural cavity, the site of mesothelioma formation" (Bernstein et al. 2010, 961). The study results were reviewed by G-P's legal team prior to publication. As questions of ghostwriting and potential fraud arose, judges and lawyers requested the original study results. G-P, now owned by Koch Industries, Inc. refused to release results on the grounds that the studies were confidential. This claim of confidentiality is bogus because true science is shared knowledge. Holm et al. were intentionally seeding the scientific literature with studies claiming that asbestos was safe. And in the meantime, workers continued to be exposed to asbestos and put at risk for lung disease and death. Manipulating study design is an ideal way to hide pseudoscience. To the non-expert, the study appears to be legitimate. The resulting confusion and chaos allow the manufacturer to continue marketing the product to unsuspecting customers.

Evaluation Design

Evaluation studies are research studies testing the process, impact, or outcome of a treatment, intervention, or program. Process evaluation looks at how feasible a program is within a particular population through attendance rates or feedback from program organizers or study participants. *Impact evaluation* looks at the short-term changes in knowledge, attitudes, or skills. *Outcome evaluation* looks at long-term changes in behavior or disease status. Evaluation studies identify evidence-based programs, practices, and treatments. Evidence-based interventions are interventions proven to work through rigorous research. Any type of the study design may be used to determine process, impact, or outcome. Qualitative methods may be used to gain process feedback on a program while true experimental or quasi-experimental methods may be used to measure impact or outcome. One dilemma of evaluation studies is how to handle the issue of the control group receiving no treatment. It seems unethical to offer no treatment to one group while the other group receives treatment. One way to get around this problem is to offer usual care, whatever intervention is currently being used to address the problem. Another solution is to provide delayed care, to offer the intervention to the control group at the end of the study. Unfortunately, researchers may become so focused on the science that they neglect to consider program participants. The Baltimore Lead Paint Study is an example of evaluation design where researchers failed to consider the potential consequences of their project.

The Baltimore Lead Paint Study

The Johns Hopkins-Kennedy Krieger Institute Baltimore Lead Paint Study is an example of the ethical challenges raised by evaluation research. Prior to 1978, lead was added to house paint to speed up drying and increase durability. Lead is a toxic metal, which damages the brain, kidneys, nerves, and blood. Lead enters the body through ingestion of peeling or flaking paint or dust. Homes built before 1978 are likely to contain leaded paint creating risk for adults and children living in the house. Children with small bodies and developing brain tissue and teething toddlers who put all kinds of things in their mouth are at high risk for lead poisoning. The average cost of full lead abatement (reducing the possibility of lead contamination) was approximately $20,000 at the time of the study. The high cost makes abatement prohibitive in low-income communities. The Repair and Maintenance Study was a study to evaluate effectiveness of different types of residential lead abatement. Johns Hopkins-Kennedy Krieger received a $200,000 grant from the Environmental Protection Agency to compare different abatement techniques. Through the program, landlords could apply for grants and loans to support lead cleanup. Selection criteria for the houses were size (800–1,200 sq. ft.), structural integrity, working utilities, not excessively furnished (to facilitate collection of dust samples), and presence of a child aged 6 months to 10 years old who spent at least 75 percent of time at the address. To participate in the program, landlords must rent to families with young children. One hundred and seven houses, 140 children were enrolled in the study. Houses were classified as Level I,

II, or III (experimental groups) or previously abated modern urban (control groups). Families were offered small tokens for study participation, such as a T-shirt or $15 for completing a survey. In addition to taking dust, soil, and water samples for lead analysis, the researchers gathered blood samples from the children at baseline and at 2, 6, 12, 18, and 24 months. The researchers did not provide families with the children's blood lead levels immediately and in some cases waited as long as nine months. Two mothers sued Kennedy Krieger for failing to provide informed consent and failing to notify parents of high lead levels. The lawsuit was initially thrown out and then overturned on appeal. In scathing criticism, Judge Dale Cathell wrote:

> It can be argued that the researchers intended that the children be the canaries in the mines but never clearly told the parents. (It was a practice in earlier years, and perhaps even now, for subsurface miners to rely on canaries to determine whether dangerous levels of toxic gases were accumulating in the mines. Canaries were particularly susceptible to such gases. When the canaries began to die, the miners knew that dangerous levels of gases were accumulating.) (*Ericka Grimes v Kennedy Krieger Institute, Inc.* No 128, September Term, 2000 and *Myron Higgins, a minor, etc., et al. v. Kennedy Krieger Institute, Inc.* No 129, September Term, 2000, 4)

Judge Cathell likened the lead paint study to the Tuskegee Syphilis Study. The study raised questions regarding parental rights to consent for children to participate in non-therapeutic research. While the study benefited communities in identifying the best practices in lead paint removal, the research did not benefit the actual study participants.

Clinical Trials

Clinical trials are a form of evaluation research. Clinical trials are research studies evaluating new drugs, medical devices, or interventions. The studies are very expensive and typically financed by industry for research and development (R&D) of new products. All clinical trials must be approved by the Food and Drug Administration (FDA). Testing a new drug or medical device proceeds in five stages:

- Phase 0 is an exploratory study testing a microdose through limited human exposure.
- Phase I tests the treatment on a small group (20–80) of healthy study volunteers in order to determine safety of the medication or device.
- Phase II studies effectiveness of the treatment over a short period of time in a larger group (i.e., 100–300) of people who have the disease or condition.

- Phase III studies effectiveness in a larger population (i.e., up to 3,000) at different dosages or in combination with other drugs.

- Phase IV occurs after the FDA has approved the treatment for use. This phase monitors safety and effectiveness.

Study 329 (chapter 3) appears to have been a Phase II clinical trial. The Comparison of Atypicals in First Episode study (chapter 2) was a Phase III clinical trial. Many pharmaceutical companies contract early clinical trials to an outside individual or contract research organization (CRO). CROs manage the space, equipment, and personnel needed to carry out clinical research studies. The researchers publish the results of the clinical trial in professional journals so that other scientists and medical practitioners can benefit from the information. The problem with corporate financing of clinical trials is how the financing influences the results. In 1997, Dr. Andrew Goudie, psychopharmacologist at University of Liverpool, requested funding from AstraZeneca for a proposed study. The Director of Clinical Science at AstraZeneca responded that Seroquel studies were no longer under the R&D Department. The studies were the responsibility of Sales and Marketing (Law Project for Psychiatric Rights n.d.). With high finances at stake, clinical trials are raising greater scrutiny. A review of clinical trials comparing antipsychotic medications found that 9 out of 10 concluded positively for the drug of the funding pharmaceutical company (Vedantam 2006). Using clinical trials as a marketing strategy jeopardizes patient care. Patients may no longer get the best possible treatment.

Survey Research

Survey research is a popular form of research in health and psychology because surveys are inexpensive and allow researchers to collect data from a large number of participants in relatively short time. Surveys can gather descriptive information on a particular population of interest, explore emerging health issues, investigate correlations, or confirm research hypotheses. The advantages of surveys are that they are inexpensive, can access large numbers of study participants, are flexible—questions may be adjusted easily, and the participant does much of the work in reading and answering the questions. Disadvantages of surveys are that the questions require standardization, information tends to be superficial, and response rates are notoriously poor. Surveys may be used as the data collection tool within many different study designs. The researcher might use a survey to assess the impact of a smoking cessation program (evaluation design) or to count physical activity after the implementation of a playground (quasi-experimental design). Surveys are also used in epidemiological research, identifying at risk groups for a particular disease or monitoring health status of large populations (see the National

Health and Nutrition Examination Survey in chapter 5). Surveys are one of the easiest and most common forms of research design.

The Hawthorne Effect

In November 1924, Western Electric Company asked industrial researcher Elton Mayo to investigate the impact of different levels of lighting on worker productivity. The electric company wanted to find ways to encourage individuals and businesses to use more electricity. The research was conducted at the Hawthorne Works plant outside of Chicago. Data were collected by Mayo's graduate assistant Fritz J. Roethlisberger with the help of William J. Dickson, director of the Department of Employee Relations at Western Electric. Results showed: (1) at higher illumination, worker productivity increased; (2) at lower illumination, worker productivity increased; and (3) productivity of the control group increased! When the study finished, productivity slumped. Mayo and Roethlisberger could not explain the results and went on to study other aspects of human behavior in the workplace. In 1958, sociologist Henry A. Landsberger reviewed Mayo's study and coined the term *the Hawthorne Effect* to describe how individuals adjust their behavior when they know they are being observed. The Hawthorne Effect is particularly relevant to research where the scientist is observing and collecting information from study volunteers. Related to the Hawthorne Effect is the idea of social desirability of participant responses. With the concept of social desirability, study volunteers give the survey response that they believe the researcher wants in a particular situation or on a survey question. Typically, social desirability is associated with socially acceptable behavior. For example, when college students take a survey on alcohol usage, they may underreport their own drinking behavior because excessive drinking carries a negative social stigma (and has many unhealthy consequences).

Unobtrusive Designs

The previously listed study designs all interact with study participants to varying degrees. With unobtrusive measures, the researcher does not interact with study participants. Data are collected through one or more secondary sources. Examples of unobtrusive measures are existing data research, content analysis, historical records, systematic reviews, and meta-analyses. Existing data research is when the researcher accesses a large database to retrieve information on the variables of interest. An example of existing data research could be accessing records of motor vehicle crashes to determine if laws banning texting while driving are associated with fewer crashes. With content analysis, the researcher reviews records maintained or collected by another individual or organization. Examples might be reviewing children's television programming to count the number of fast food advertisements that children are exposed to or reviewing patient charts to identify physician screening for intimate partner violence. Historical records are books, exhibits, reports, or other evidence that represents a particular moment in history. An example of historical research might be a review of cigarette advertising throughout the twentieth century to track marketing trends. Systematic review is an advanced type of literature review. The researcher collects, reads, and analyzes selected sources of information in order to answer a research question. A meta-analysis is similar to a systematic review except the researcher summarizes the original sources by statistical analysis. The advantage of unobtrusive measures is that the researcher does not encounter the Hawthorne Effect. Reviewing past records allows the researcher to cover a broad expanse of time, something that may not be possible through one single study. These are also fairly inexpensive studies because the data have already been collected and recorded. Unobtrusive measures offer high replicability. If the researcher makes a mistake, it is possible to go back and re-examine the source. Disadvantages are that unobtrusive research is not rich in details and the information may not have been recorded accurately, some information may not be recorded at all, or is not recorded in a way that the researcher can use. With unobtrusive research design, the researcher can only access what is available.

There are many different ways to study a topic. Research designs provide a blueprint for a study. The researcher must select the best design based on time, resources, access to study participants, and purpose of the study. Unfortunately, there is no perfect study design and the researcher must weigh the advantages and disadvantages of each type of design in order to come up with the best fit. Just like other steps in the scientific method, it is easy for unscrupulous individuals to manipulate study design to support a particular agenda.

FURTHER READING

Bernstein, D. M., R. A. Rogers, R. Sepulveda, K. Donaldson, D. Schuler, S. Gaering, P. Kunzendorf, J. Chevalier, and S. E. Holm. 2010. "The Pathological Response and Fate in the Lung and Pleura of Chrysotile in Combination with Fine Particles Compared to Amosite Asbestos Following Short-Term Inhalation Exposure: Interim Results." *Inhalation Toxicology* 22 (11): 937–62.

Bernstein, David M., K. Donaldson, U. Decker, S. Gaering, P. Kunzendorf, J. Chevalier, and S. E. Holm. 2008. "A Biopersistence Study following Exposure to Chrysotile Asbestos Alone or in Combination with Fine Particles." *Inhalation Toxicology* 20 (11): 1009–28.

Cooke, W. E. 1924. "Fibrosis of the Lungs due to the Inhalation of Asbestos Dust." *British Medical Journal* 2 (3317): 147.

Doll, R., and A. B. Hill. 1954. "The Mortality of Doctors in Relation to Their Smoking Habits." *British Medical Journal* 1 (4877): 1451–1455.

Dominus, Susan. 2011. "The Crash and Burn of an Autism Guru." *The New York Times Magazine*, April 20. Accessed January 17, 2018. https://www.nytimes.com/2011/04/24/magazine/mag-24Autism-t.html

Ericka Grimes v. Kennedy Krieger Institute, Inc. No 128, September Term, 2000 and *Myron Higgins, a minor, etc., et al. v. Kennedy Krieger Institute, Inc.* No 129, September Term, 2000. Accessed August 18, 2019. https://courts.state.md.us/data/opinions/coa/2001/128a00.pdf

Fleischer, Walter E., Frederick J. Viles, Robert L. Gade, and Philip Drikker. 1946. "A Health Survey of Pipe Covering Operations in Constructing Naval Vessels." *Journal of Industrial Hygiene and Toxicology* 28 (1): 9–16.

Freed, Gary L., Sarah J. Clark, Amy T. Butchart, Dianne C. Singer, and Matthew M. Davis. 2010. "Parental Vaccine Safety Concerns in 2009." *Pediatrics* 125 (4): 654–59.

Humphreys, Laud. 1970. "Tearoom Trade: Impersonal Sex in Public Places." *Trans-Action: Social Science & Modern Society* 7 (3): 10–25.

Landsberger, Henry A. 1958. *Hawthorne Revisited: Management and the Worker: Its Critics, and Developments in Human Relations in Industry.* Cornell Studies in Industrial and Labor Relations, vol. 9. Ithaca, NY: Cornell University Press.

Law Project for Psychiatric Rights. n.d. "AstraZeneca Corporate Witness and Key Opinion Leader Deposition Exhibits." Accessed August 18, 2019. http://psychrights.org/Research/Digest/NLPs/Seroquel/090520UnsealedSeroquelExhibits/DocumentDescriptionTables.pdf

Morris, Jim. 2013. "Facing Lawsuits over Deadly Asbestos, Paper Giant Launched Secretive Research Program." The Center for Public Integrity. Accessed May 5, 2018. https://www.publicintegrity.org/2013/10/21/13559/facing-lawsuits-over-deadly-asbestos-paper-giant-launched-secretive-research

Public Health England. 2014. "Confirmed Cases of Measles, Mumps and Rubella 1996–2013." *The National Archives*. Accessed January 17, 2019. https://webarchive.nationalarchives.gov.uk/20140505192923/http://www.hpa.org.uk/web/HPAweb&HPAwebStandard/HPAweb_C/1195733833790

Spriggs, M. 2004. "Canaries in the Mines: Children, Risk, Non-Therapeutic Research, and Justice." *Journal of Medical Ethics* 30 (2): 176–81.

U.S. Environmental Protection Agency. 1996. "Lead-based Paint Abatement and Repair and Maintenance Study in Baltimore: Pre-intervention Findings." Accessed June 1, 2019. https://www.epa.gov/sites/production/files/documents/r95-012.pdf

Vedantam, Shankar. 2006. "Comparison of Schizophrenia Drugs Often Favors Firm Funding Study." *Washington Post*, April 12. Accessed January 24, 2018. https://www.washingtonpost.com/archive/politics/2006/04/12/comparison-of-schizophrenia-drugs-often-favors-firm-funding-study/b97b328b-07c1-4f28-95c9-04d137a072d1/

Vigen, Tyler. 2015. "Spurious Correlations." Accessed January 24, 2018. http://www.tylervigen.com/spurious-correlations

Wakefield, A. J., S. H. Murch, A. Anthony, J. Linnell, D. M. Casson, M. Malik, M. Berelowitz, et al. 1998. "Retracted: Ileal-Lymphoid-Nodular Hyperplasia, Non-Specific Colitis, and Pervasive Developmental Disorder in Children." *The Lancet* 351 (9103): 637–41.

FIVE

Study Sample

Collecting scientific data is costly and time-consuming. To control expenses and ensure efficient use of resources, researchers use sampling, the technique of collecting data from a carefully selected smaller group. In theory, the sample should exhibit the same characteristics or attributes as the larger population of interest. Sampling allows the researcher to draw conclusions about the population of interest without collecting data from every person or item in the population. In health and psychology, the study sample is often human beings. However, researchers may also collect data from mice, dogs, body tissue, patient charts, census records, occupational health reports, or other sources. The group that participates in the study is known as the study sample or sample population. The larger group is the theoretical population or target population. The individual units that the researcher collects data from are study elements. The National Health and Nutrition Examination Survey (NHANES) provides an example of how these concepts apply in practice. NHANES is a survey that investigates the health, nutrition, and physical activity of children and adults in the United States. The survey includes in-home interviews and clinical examination of height, weight, blood pressure, bone density, eyesight, kidney function, sexually transmitted diseases, blood tests, and other physiological functions. It would be impossible and extraordinarily expensive to collect data on every person in America to get an accurate picture of the health status of Americans. Researchers collect data from a sample of 5,000 randomly selected people. Each of the 5,000 study participants represents another 50,000 people. Collecting data from 5,000 people is more realistic and achievable than collecting data from 250 million people. The NHANES data provide interesting and valuable information. The height and weight charts that pediatricians use to screen children for developmental delays, malnutrition, or overweight were developed from the NHANES survey results. Health professionals use NHANES data to track obesity rates throughout the nation and to plan programs based on regional health needs. Using a smaller group of people to represent the larger population of American citizens ensures that health resources are used wisely and where they are most needed. Study samples allow researchers to collect information, test hypotheses, and draw accurate conclusions about the theoretical population within reasonable time and resource constraints.

Ideally, the research goal is to gather a study sample that matches the theoretical population. There are times when the researcher fails and the sample population does not adequately reflect the theoretical population. The classic example of study sample-theoretical population mismatch is the case of the once-popular journal *Literary Digest*. In 1916, 1920, 1924, 1928, and 1932, the *Literary Digest* successfully predicted the outcome of each presidential election. In 1936, the magazine created a survey to predict the winner of the presidential race between Kansas Governor Alfred Landon and incumbent President Franklin Delano Roosevelt. This would be the *Literary Digest*'s largest survey ever. Staff gathered names from magazine subscriptions, telephone directories, and automobile registrations. Survey administrators sent surveys to 10 million people. Even by today's standards, this is a huge study sample. Over 2 million people responded. Survey results indicated that Landon would win by a landslide. Roosevelt won. With the benefit of hindsight, the *Literary Digest* successfully predicted who wealthy voters would elect, not who the American public would elect. The *Literary Digest* sampled people who could afford magazines, cars, and telephones, people with higher income. Roosevelt was elected as the nation was recovering from the Great Depression. Roosevelt's New Deal promised federal aid programs, recovery, and support for working-class voters. The *Literary Digest* never regained their reputation as a credible news source and eventually went out of business.

By definition, a sample is a representative part of a greater whole or group. The purpose of sampling is representation. One strange case where the researcher simply did not seem to understand this concept is that of Maria Cristina Miron Elqutub. Elqutub was investigating salivary gland carcinoma risk among genetic variants at the University of Texas MD Anderson Cancer Center. As part of the study procedures, Elqutub was to collect blood from patients. Instead, she used her own blood and labeled the samples as belonging to 98 different patients. The substitution came out when another study team at MD Anderson looked at the samples for a different study. They quickly realized that the samples did not vary. They were not actually samples. Elqutub had published her study in two research papers on salivary gland carcinomas. Both papers were retracted by the publishers. After investigation by the Office of Research Integrity, Elqutub voluntarily agreed to attain institutional supervision of her research for a period of three years and to exclude herself from volunteering in any service or advisory capacity with the U.S. Public Health Service. At last report, Elqutub was working as a school nurse in a middle school. She never gave a reason for not collecting the blood samples.

Sampling errors are flaws in study results that occur when the study sample does not reflect the theoretical population. The Louise Wise Services study of twins and triplets separated at birth is another example of flawed sample design (chapter 2). The study was supposed to investigate nature vs. nurture among children with the same genetic makeup. Twins and triplets from multiparous births can be either monozygotic or dizygotic. Monozygotic twins are genetically identical because the babies develop from the same sperm and egg. Dizygotic twins or fraternal twins develop from separate eggs and separate sperm cells. Neubauer and co-investigators never verified genetic makeup to ensure identicalness of the study participants. Study participants were never screened to see if they were identical or fraternal. The researchers assumed that all of the twins and the triplets were monozygotic. Sampling errors can lead to skewed results and faulty conclusions. Therefore, researchers go to great lengths to ensure that the study sample matches the theoretical population.

In some studies, the inability to generalize to the theoretical population is simply a limitation of the study. For example, the Youth Risk Behavior Surveillance System (YRBSS) is a survey of health behaviors by the Centers for Disease Control and Prevention (CDC). The survey collects information on intentional and unintentional injuries, substance abuse, sexuality, diet, physical activity, and other health behaviors in order to identify current health issues and trends experienced by America's young people. Through agreements with local organizations and schools and with permission from parents, surveys are administered to students attending randomly selected high schools across the nation. The data are used by federal, state, and local health officials to set public priorities, determine funding, plan programs, and define health goals of the nation. In 2017, usable data were collected from 14,765 students (U.S. Department of Health and Human Services 2018). Despite the large number of respondents, one major limitation of the survey is that the procedures survey youth in school. Approximately 5 percent of youth who are eligible to attend high school are not registered or attending. Youth may be absent due to chronic illness, addiction, homelessness, violence, or other health-related obstacles. If youth missing school are in poorer health than those in school, the true incidence and prevalence rates of risky health behaviors may be higher than the data provided by the YRBSS. Yet, it would be expensive and nearly impossible to track down missing or absent youth and survey each individually. As a result, the YRBSS is not 100 percent reflective of all youth in the United States. Despite limitations, the survey gives sufficient information for strategic health planning.

SAMPLING DESIGNS AND SAMPLING METHODS

Sampling designs are the plan of how the researcher hopes to attain a representative sample. Sampling methods are the actual procedures that researchers use to attain the sample. The first step in creating a study sample is to define the theoretical population. In the case of NHANES, the theoretical population is all adults and children in the United States. The researcher then works backward, identifying possible filters that may limit generalizability. With NHANES, a random sample of U.S. residents may not include enough older adults, African American, Asian, and Hispanic Americans to adequately reflect these minority populations. To compensate for underrepresentation, researchers may oversample some groups. NHANES uses a multistep sampling design. In Stage 1, all counties in the United States are categorized into 15 groups according to certain characteristics. One county is selected from each group. Stage 2 divides the 15 counties into smaller sampling segments, focusing on households as opposed to parks or shopping districts. Approximately 20 of the sampling segments are randomly selected from each of the 15 counties. In Stage 3, the sampling segments are divided up by households and a sample of about 30 households is selected from each of the sampling segments. NHANES researchers visit each of the selected households and collect basic information on all of the residents in the household. In Stage 4, a computer randomly selects the final study participants from the list of people identified by the household visits. In theory, each and every American adult and child has an equal and probable chance of selection to participate in the NHANES survey. This concept is referred to as EPSEM, equal probability of selection method sampling. EPSEM reduces sampling error. There is a stronger chance that the study sample reflects the theoretical population and study findings are generalizable.

Researchers use different procedures and techniques to define and develop their study sample. The two main types of sampling methods are probability and nonprobability sampling. Probability sampling uses the concept of EPSEM. Study participants or study elements are randomly drawn from a list of the larger population. Putting names in a basket and randomly drawing the names from the basket is a form of probability sampling. Asking people to count by fives and then taking every fifth person is another example of probability sampling. There are several different methods of probability sampling to help the researcher attain a representative study sample. If the researcher knows that random selection could lead to underrepresented groups, the researcher may divide participants based on that attribute and then oversample the underrepresented groups. Recruitment becomes more complicated when the researcher intends to study behaviors or groups with unusual characteristics. Nonprobability sampling is a form of sampling where the researcher purposely selects participants based on a particular attribute or experience. For example, if the researcher wants to study substance abuse among physicians, the researcher needs to recruit doctors with a current or past history of substance abuse. Random sampling of a group of physicians would not work. Many of the interviewees may not have abused illicit substances and would not be able to describe experiences. Advertising for study participants with the American Medical Association is also unlikely to work. Few doctors would be willing to risk their license or professional standing to participate in the study. The researcher could use a type of nonprobability known as snowball sampling method. With snowball sampling, the researcher identifies one or two individuals, in this case doctors who abuse or formerly abused substances. The initial participants refer other participants who then refer subsequent participants. The sample grows through building trust and word of mouth referrals. Snowball sampling is good for exploring private topics, personal information that people may not wish to discuss openly, or when the study population may be difficult to identify and recruit. The disadvantage of nonprobability sampling is that study results cannot be generalized to the larger group.

CONVENIENCE SAMPLES

Recruiting human study participants is challenging. The ideal study participant is responsible, able to follow study procedures, and willing to report any adverse experiences resulting from study participation. By their nature, responsible people are busy with other obligations. They may not have the time or motivation to take part in a research study. On the other hand, a researcher cannot force people to fill out a survey or take part in an experiment because that would be unethical, a violation of human participant protections. To overcome obstacles in recruiting, researchers in education, sociology, psychology, and health often partner with schools, hospitals, community organizations, or other institutions that offer potential access to study participants. Students at school, elderly in a nursing home, members of a club, homeless people, inmates in prison, or people in the workplace are often perceived as easily accessible study samples or convenience samples. Convenience samples raise several concerns. The first issue is coercion. Is the researcher respecting participant autonomy? Is there an assumption that services or assistance may be denied if individuals prefer not to participate? Do individuals feel comfortable in refusing to participate in the study? The second issue relates to generalizability. How well does the study sample reflect the theoretical sample? The use of a convenience sample makes it easy for researchers to miss the bigger picture of whom or where they are collecting data. Researchers may become so focused on data collection that they miss important ethical or scientific considerations.

College students are a common convenience sample (Hanel and Vione 2016). Professors can administer their survey in the classroom, eliminating the need and cost of laboratory space, and students are more likely to complete the entire survey because they are conditioned to answer questions in the classroom. The Stanford Prison Experiment described in chapter 6 is an example of college students as study participants. Almost 90 percent of consumer research studies use college students as study participants (Peterson 2001). However, there are limitations to the use of college students in research and overrepresentation of college students can be problematic. As a demographic, college students tend to be younger, more intellectually curious, conscientious, and motivated to achieve life goals. They also tend to be from higher socioeconomic levels than nonstudents and have less experience in the day-to-day struggles of young adults. Thus, college students are appropriate for theory research, where the researchers are attempting to develop a theory. They are less appropriate for effects application research, where the researcher is attempting to discover attitudes, experiences, or behavior of young people. Personal attributes can vary based on the student's major course of study. Psychology students demonstrate attitudes that are more benevolent while business students value power (Bardi et al. 2014). In terms of overrepresentation of students in research, the amount of literature written and published on a topic is an indirect indicator of how important that issue is. With college students as easily accessible study participants, more literature might appear on an issue such as test anxiety than on Alzheimer's disease. Certain problems may be more highly represented in the literature. A final issue for scientists considering students as convenient study participants is the ethical principle of respect for persons. According to Milgram's Conditions of Authority, when an adult in a position of authority distributes a survey in class, students may feel obligated to complete the survey. There is a sense of underlying coercion. Furthermore, students attend school to learn. They do not attend school to serve as study participants. Collecting data in schools may interfere with the learning process and the researcher must consider whether study participation is really in the best interest of the students.

With global commerce and increased recognition of the interconnectedness of health, international samples grow in popularity. This is a good thing. Pathogens do not respect borders or political boundaries. There is a need to study and contain infectious diseases at the source of outbreak. Cultural exchange also introduces diseases that were once exclusive to specific countries. For example, America has done a great job at exporting our love of fast food and with it, the problem of obesity. As international research expands, the issue of *ethics dumping* emerged (see chapter 2). Ethics dumping is a term coined by the European Commission describing the practice where researchers from high-income countries do research in low- or middle-income countries in order to circumvent ethics review. The researcher knows that lower income countries do not have the resources to review and monitor studies and they may be able to get away with practices considered unethical in more regulated countries with sufficient resources to monitor human participant protections.

Historically, prisons were considered an easy source of study participants for research. During the eighteenth century, some prisoners in the United Kingdom were given the option of being hanged or exposed to smallpox. Scottish physician and scientist Andre Ure performed gruesome experiments on executed prisoners. In 1818, Ure attempted to revive Matthew Clydesdale after he was executed by hanging. Ure stimulated the phrenic nerve causing Clydesdale's body to convulse and grimace. The experiment was stopped when Ure's terrorized audience ran out. By the mid-1970s, 85 percent of Phase 1 clinical trials were conducted on prisoners (Charles et al. 2016). Using prisoners as study participants benefits the pharmaceutical company, the prison, and, if the study is benign, the inmates. Pharmaceutical research reduces the cost of medical care in prisons. Qualified research staff can provide much needed medical care to inmates volunteering for studies. Clinical research studies can relieve some of the boredom of prison and offer small payments for the purchase of personal items or cigarettes. Pharmaceutical companies benefit by having numerous bodies to test the steady stream of drugs in development. One obstacle to using inmates as study subjects is transporting prisoners from the prison to the clinical research unit. To overcome this obstacle, many clinical research units were established within prisons. The business relationship between pharmaceutical companies and prisons combined with the lack of autonomy and education of the inmates creates a huge imbalance of power where prisoners may be easily taken advantage of. The case of Albert Kligman's dermatological studies show how money, status, and vulnerability do not mix well in research.

Dr. Albert Kligman and Retin-A

Dermatologist Dr. Albert Kligman first visited Philadelphia's Holmesburg Prison in 1951 to investigate an outbreak of athlete's foot. The former botanist recalled hundreds of men roaming around shirtless in the heat of the summer and envisioned "acres of skin" to test his experimental skin products (Hornblum 1998). The prison conditions were ideal for a highly controlled laboratory. Skin creams, deodorant, shampoo, foot powders, and hair dye could be applied, tested, and retested. Creating a grid with adhesive tape on the study participant's back, one study participant could test up to 20 formulas at once. Kligman and other researchers at the University of Pennsylvania paid $10 per section of skin, significantly more than the 15–25 cents a day for prison duties. The tests included exposing the applied substance to a heat lamp at varying temperatures. Researchers assessed degree of burning, peeling, or blistering. Although, the skin tests were painful and sometimes left permanent scars, the men were a captive, uneducated audience with little else to do during incarceration. Through the studies and his easy access to study participants, Kligman became a highly regarded dermatologist. Dow Chemical paid him $10,000 to test dioxin, the main toxin in Agent Orange. Kligman discovered Retin-A, a medication to treat acne, wrinkles, and sun-damaged skin. Retin-A made Kligman a very wealthy man.

Allen M. Hornblum joined Holmesburg prison staff in 1971 working as the director of the adult literacy program. He was curious about the gauze patches that many men wore on their backs. He knew that the men were poorly educated and may not understand the long-term effects of experimental chemicals. Within a year, the story of the Tuskegee Syphilis Study broke raising concerns about the abuse of vulnerable populations in research. Hornblum and ethicists began to question studies on prisoners. The dermatological studies ended in 1974. Hornblum documented the prisoners' experiences in his books *Acres of Skin* and *Sentenced to Science*. Kligman defended the studies noting that they were done at a time when informed consent and human participant protections were not as refined as they are now.

Today, ethics committees are particularly careful in reviewing and approving research on prisoners. U.S. and UK scientists may only perform research on prisoners if the purpose of the study specifically relates to the prison population. In 2014, a review of 14,355 applications for studies in England and Wales found that only 100 studies (0.7 percent) proposed prisoners as study participants (Charles et al. 2016). The main reasons for not including prisoners in research are logistical, ethical, and scientific. Logistically, it is difficult to manage study participants who are incarcerated without setting up a lab in the prison. Scientifically, prisoners may not be representative of other populations of interest. Generalizability is reduced. The lack of studies among prisoners now raises a question of the impact on inmate health. Prisoners have higher rates of substance abuse, mental illness, and communicable disease. Does the new protectionist approach negatively impact prisoner health?

SELECTION OF STUDY PARTICIPANTS

The study sample is defined prior to the start of the study. Naming the sample ensures that the researchers clearly define who will be included and who will be excluded from the study. Inclusion criteria are the characteristics necessary for participation in the study. Typical inclusion criteria are related to demographics, clinical criteria (presence of disease or disorder), or geographic location. Exclusion criteria are additional characteristics that disqualify someone who meets the inclusion criteria. Exclusion criteria are typically factors that restrict participation or increase risk of an adverse event, such as presence of one or more comorbidities, inability to follow study directions (problems with literacy or substance abuse), or inability to attend appointments. In the Comparison of Atypicals in First Episode study (chapter 2), inclusion criteria were:

- Males and females ages 16–40 years with schizophreniform disorder, schizophrenia, or schizoaffective disorder.
- Psychotic symptoms lasting for at least one month and no more than five years.
- No history of previous treatment with antipsychotics for more than 16 weeks.

Exclusion criteria were:

- Patients with a history of recovery lasting three months or more.
- Pregnant or nursing females.
- Patients with mental retardation.
- Patients who are suicidal.

Inclusion and exclusion criteria are important in ensuring human participant protections and generalizability of the study results. The cases of Drs. Roger Poisson and Mani Pavuluri highlight the importance of defining and adhering to clear inclusion and exclusion criteria.

Dr. Roger Poisson and the National Surgical Adjuvant Breast and Bowel Project

In 1975, Dr. Roger Poisson joined Saint Luc Hospital working on the National Surgical Adjuvant Breast and Bowel Project (NSABP). Poisson directed the research team and worked as professor of surgery at the University of Montreal. The NSABP started in 1958 as collaboration between U.S. and Canadian doctors comparing the effectiveness of various breast cancer treatments. By the early 1990s, over 5,000 patients from 485 hospitals participated in the study. The Saint Luc study team worked on several protocols. Protocol B-6 compared the effectiveness of lumpectomy (removal of the tumor) plus radiation vs. full mastectomy (removal of the breast). Based on the results of Protocol B-6, doctors moved away from recommending full mastectomy to patients with breast cancer. Protocol 13 compared the disease-free survival rates of patients with estrogen-receptor-negative (ER-) breast tumors who received no treatment and patients who received a sequential combination of methotrexate to Flouracil. Protocol 14 assessed the survival rates with tamoxifen vs. no treatment. Protocol B-16 compared tamoxifen alone and two other combinations of drugs with tamoxifen. The inclusion and exclusion criteria for the study were complex. For example, the selection criteria for Protocol B-6 were women with operable breast cancer and the primary tumor had to be 4 cm or less in dimension and movable (not adhering to the skin, muscle, or chest wall). There could be no evidence of skin or lymph node involvement

unless the lymph nodes were also moveable. The breast tissue had to be of sufficient size to allow cosmetic removal. Study participants were randomly assigned
to treatment groups. Between 1977 and 1991, Saint Luc Hospital accounted for 16
percent of all NSABP study participants.

While checking Protocol B-16 data, the NSABP statistician discovered two
different copies of study reports on the same Saint Luc Hospital patient. All of
the information was identical except the date of surgery. One copy made the
patient eligible for the study. The other copy reported a longer time between the
date of the operation and date of randomization. In September 1990, the deputy
director of the NSABP Biostatistical Center performed a routine site visit at Saint
Luc Hospital and followed up on the discrepancy. He concluded that there was no
intentional deception. The researchers seemed to misunderstand selection criteria. The site monitor recommended further audit. In early 1991, three NSABP
staff visited Saint Luc and reviewed 120 charts of patients in the Protocol B-18
study and random records of study participants in eight other protocols. The team
found five alterations to the records. The NSABP suspended studies at Saint Luc
Hospital and notified the funder, the National Cancer Institute (NCI). The Office
of Research Integrity investigated and found 115 cases of data fabrication or falsification. Most of the alterations enhanced study eligibility by adjusting the dates
of biopsy or surgery or hormone receptor values. Poisson admitted falsifying the
data. He kept two sets of records, one marked "true" and one marked "false."
While the investigation was ongoing, statisticians reanalyzed published data.
They were concerned with the impact the data may have on women seeking treatment for breast cancer. Multiple reanalysis found similar results to the original
study. Poisson's manipulation did not change the study results. Public notice of
the research misconduct was released in spring 1993 and the telephone lines at
the American Cancer Society were flooded with calls. The delay between discovery of the scientific misconduct and the final investigative report raised concerns
that scientists were covering up mistakes.

After full investigation, the Office of Research Integrity discovered Poisson
had falsified medical records of 99 of the patients. He was banned from serving
on Public Health Service advisory board or review committees and from receiving U.S. government research funding for eight years. In his defense, Poisson
explained:

> I felt that the rules were meant to be understood as guidelines and not nec-
> essarily followed blindly. My sole concern at all times was the health of my
> patients. I firmly believed that a patient who was able to enter into a NASBP
> trial received the best therapy and follow-up treatment. For me, it was dif-
> ficult to tell a woman with breast cancer that she was ineligible to receive
> the best available treatment because she did not meet 1 criterion out of 22,
> when I knew that this criterion had little or no intrinsic oncologic impor-
> tance. (Fisher and Redmond 1994, 1460)

Poisson retired from his position at the University of Montreal on April 30, 1993. The NSABP studies continue to seek the most effective methods of breast cancer treatment and prevention.

Dr. Mani Pavuluri and Bipolar Children

Dr. Mani Pavuluri was a preeminent child psychiatrist and professor of psychiatry at the University of Illinois at Chicago (UIC) specializing in the diagnosis and treatment of mood-related disorders among children. Her achievements included authoring a handbook entitled *What Works for Bipolar Kids: Help and Hope for Parents*, securing approximately $7.5 million in federal grant funding, recognition as one of the most prominent women in child psychiatry, and honored as a distinguished fellow by the American Academy of Child and Adolescent Psychiatry. Pavuluri was a major draw for UIC's Pediatric Mood Disorders Program attracting over a thousand patients to the clinic. In 2009, the nationally recognized psychiatrist designed a study to assess the use of lithium as treatment for bipolar disorder in adolescents. Bipolar disorder is also known as manic-depressive illness. The disorder is characterized by extreme changes in mood, energy, and activity levels. The individual swings from periods of deep depression to extreme mania over a period of days or weeks. Manic periods can include severe sleeplessness, hallucinations, rage, psychosis, or paranoia. Lithium effectively stabilizes mood in adults with bipolar disorder. Less is known about the effects of lithium in children or the impact of the drug on the developing brain. Pavuluri's study proposed taking images of brain activity during a manic state and again after eight weeks on lithium and comparing these images to the brain scans of healthy volunteers. The National Institute of Mental Health (NIMH) initially rejected Pavuluri's request for funding due to safety concerns with the use of lithium in children. Pavuluri revised the proposal to exclude children younger than 13 years of age and the NIMH approved $3.1 million of funding for the study. In addition to the age restriction, the NIMH insisted on the following criteria:

- All study participants had to be under the care and monitoring of an independent medical professional. Pavuluri could not act as both researcher and clinical psychiatrist for study participants.

- Participants could not have previously used psychotropic medications because combining lithium with psychotropic drugs is known to cause adverse effects.

- All female participants had to be screened for pregnancy to prevent fetal defects due to lithium.

UIC's IRB approved the study without seeing the full protocol. Four months after initial IRB approval, Pavuluri submitted an IRB amendment requesting that the age limit be reduced to 10 years. The IRB approved the amendment without consulting the NIMH. Pavuluri and one of her co-investigators were members of the trial's Data Safety and Monitoring Board, a committee responsible for overseeing the safety of study participants. One hundred and three study participants with bipolar disorder and 132 healthy volunteers were enrolled in the study. Pavuluri enrolled her own sons as healthy volunteers and signed their consent forms. Scientists typically do not include family members as study participants, even as healthy volunteers.

Ten-year-old Luke Mallard was having problems at school. He was defiant and acting out. His mother had tried to get an appointment with Pavuluri without success. Then she learned that signing Luke into the study would enable access to the highly respected child psychiatrist. Luke enrolled in the study. Soon after starting lithium, he exhibited signs of psychosis. He paced, walked in circles, and experienced auditory and visual hallucinations. Luke's mother finally asked Pavuluri to stop the lithium. Meanwhile, UIC had received other reports of concerns about the study. One study participant ended up in the hospital with severe irritability and aggression after Pavuluri had tried to wean her off her medications in order to enter her in the lithium study. The IRB reported the hospitalization to the Office of Human Research Protections. Two months later, university officials suspended the lithium study and two of Pavuluri's other studies. The IRB raised concerns about failure to adhere to the study protocol.

NIMH investigation revealed that 89 of the 103 study participants did not meet the study's inclusion criteria. Pavuluri tested lithium on children younger than 10, included children who had previously been on psychotropic medication, neglected to warn parents of the drug's risk, failed to inform parents of alternative treatments, failed to screen female participants for pregnancy, acted in dual roles as clinical psychiatrist and researcher, and falsified study data to cover up misconduct. During the investigation, the university continued to promote Pavuluri as a preeminent child psychiatrist. UIC recognized her with a $30,000 award for excellence in research. The NIMH concluded that Pavuluri was in serious noncompliance with human participant protections, a violation of grant funding. The federal investigators criticized UIC's IRB for failing to provide sufficient oversight and rebuked the university for continuing to promote Pavuluri's status as an expert even when they were aware of possible misconduct. The university was required to return $3.1 million of Pavuluri's research grants. In 2015, the university chancellor concluded that Pavuluri consistently placed her research above patient welfare (Cohen 2018b). In her defense, Pavuluri claimed that her mistakes were oversights and the university did not provide adequate training in research. Pavuluri resigned from her position at the university and opened a private medical practice in Chicago.

NONREPRESENTATIVE STUDY SAMPLES

Nonrepresentative samples are small or nondiverse samples that do not reflect the larger population of interest. Nonrepresentative samples are used routinely in case studies and qualitative studies. Nonrepresentative sample designs are acceptable when the researcher does not wish to generalize the results to a larger population. An important issue with small, nonrepresentative samples is that they may lead researchers to erroneous conclusions. One example of faulty conclusion based on a nonrepresentative sample is the Memorial Sloan Kettering Cancer Center pain management study by Drs. Russell K. Portenoy and Kathleen M. Foley. Portenoy and Foley followed 38 patients who were prescribed opioids for nonmalignant pain. Twelve patients were prescribed oxycodone, seven received methadone, five treated with levorphanol and the remaining patients were treated with a combination of drugs. The pain management specialists reported that only two patients developed drug dependence and these two patients had a previous history of dependence. The overall study conclusion was that opioids are safe and effective in managing pain. Pharmaceutical companies jumped at the experts' conclusions. Purdue Pharma distributed 15,000 copies of a patient education video marketing OxyContin. The video was played in doctors' waiting rooms around the nation. Within a year, the number of opioid prescriptions increased by 11 million. Today, opioid abuse is a serious public health problem. The crisis started with one small nonrepresentative sample. The 38 patients in Portenoy and Foley's study were under careful monitoring and did not represent people in the community. The Little Albert Experiment is another well-known example of a nonrepresentative study sample.

Little Albert

In the 1920s, Johns Hopkins psychologist John Broadus Watson and graduate student Rosalie Alberta Raynor studied human behavior and conditioned responses. Watson believed that he could condition infants to fear a neutral stimulus. His hypothesis was based on Pavlov's theories of classical conditioning. Pavlov conditioned dogs to salivate when they heard a bell. Watson and Raynor wondered if they could condition humans and if the emotional response would transfer to neutral objects. The study sample consisted of one infant, nine-month-old Albert B. Watson (a pseudonym). Raynor described Albert as a normal, healthy, and unemotional infant. The researchers accessed Albert through his mother, a wet nurse at Harriet Lane Hospital, part of Johns Hopkins Hospital. To determine Albert's baseline emotional reactions, the researchers exposed him to a white rat, a rabbit, a dog, a monkey, various masks, and cotton wool. Albert showed no signs of fear and attempted to reach out and touch some of the objects. To condition the response, Raynor showed Albert the white rat. As soon as Albert reached for the rat, Watson struck a steel bar with a hammer behind the child. The noise surprised Albert causing him to startle and tremble. The researchers repeated the exercise. Albert's reaction grew stronger. In some instances, he fell over or cried. By the seventh simulation, Albert withdrew when he saw the rat. The researchers repeated the procedure of exposing Albert to a rabbit, dog, monkey, and cotton wool followed by the same loud noise. Albert displayed varying reactions and the researchers concluded that emotional transfer does occur.

The Little Albert Experiment is often cited for ethical concerns. Based on her job, historians suspect the Albert's mother was a poor, single mother. Records indicate that Watson paid mothers $1 to allow him to experiment with their child (Beck, Levinson, and Irons 2009). As a scientist, Watson would have been at the higher echelon of the Johns Hopkins social hierarchy. A single mother and her child would have been lower socioeconomic class. This raises questions of whether Watson was taking advantage of a vulnerable family. A second ethical issue is that the research stopped when Albert was one year old. Mother and child moved away from Baltimore. The researchers never deconditioned the fear response. The long-term implications of the experiment are unknown. Soon after publishing the study, Watson left Hopkins. He was forced out of academia by a very public divorce involving an affair with Raynor. After leaving academia, Watson took a job in advertising where he was very successful. What is interesting is the impact of the Little Albert study on the field of classical conditioning. Despite the sample size of one and complete lack of generalizability, the Little Albert Experiment became the foundation for behaviorism. Watson is listed among the top 25 most frequently cited psychologists in introductory psychology textbooks (Haggbloom et al. 2002). The American Psychological Association awarded him a gold medal in 1957 for contributions to the discipline.

RESEARCH SUBJECTS AS GUINEA PIGS

Biomedical researchers use guinea pigs extensively in laboratory experiments. Besides being cute and adorable, the little mammals are easy to maintain, do not object to being caged, and biologically have many similarities to humans. The cavy is also particularly prone to infection making it a great specimen for studying communicable diseases. When Robert Koch had difficulty finding a cure for tuberculosis, he turned to guinea pigs to simulate human infection. Unfortunately, he prematurely announced his discovery of a cure for the Great White Plague and created overwhelming demand, frustration, and eventually anger toward scientists. In *The Quintessence of Ibsenism*, playwright George Bernard Shaw gave voice to the public disdain for science by using the guinea pig as a metaphor for human subjects' research. The term *guinea pig* continues to be used today, often by study volunteers themselves. *Guinea Pig Zero* is a webzine for people who make a job out of volunteering for medical or pharmaceutical research. Under the statement of purpose, the Guinea Pig Zero website notes, "This journal keeps in mind that we volunteers can and should maintain an awareness and a will, because if we do not, we will fall victim to the evil uses devised for us by scientists who forget that we and they are of the same species" (Guinea Pig Zero 2019). The image of study subjects as guinea pigs creates an image of use, abuse, and disregard for the rights and welfare of participants. Participants become nothing more than laboratory rats to be poked, prodded, and subjected to procedures for the purported benefit of science. There is no regard for the animal. Chapter 2 describes many cases of violations of human participant protections and the need for protections of human study participants. The Human Radiation Experiments are further examples of how elite researchers took advantage of men, women, and children using the study participants as guinea pigs in scientific experiments.

Human Radiation Experiments

During World War I, large numbers of women went to work in factories filling positions vacated by men called to battle. The U.S. Radium Corporation (USRC) recruited workers to paint luminous dials on watches and military equipment. The job required small, steady hands and paid three times the average factory job. Many of the workers were young petite teenage girls recruited by friends and family members also working in the factory. At the end of the workday, the girls glowed in the dark from the iridescent paint. They became known locally as the ghost girls. The girls embraced the label. They painted their fingernails, face, and teeth with the radium. Some wore their best party dresses to work so that the dress glowed in the dark dance hall at night. USRC managers knew that radium was hazardous. The owners and company scientists avoided exposure. Factory chemists wore lead aprons, masks, and tongs to handle the radioactive material. The girls were not given any protective equipment or informed of the hazards of exposure. As part of the training, factory supervisors told the girls to use their lips to straighten the bristles of the paintbrush when it lost point. Thus, the workers were trained to put the radium directly into their mouths. By 1925, several of the workers died from necrosis of the jaw and bone tumors. USRC denied workers' claims that the radium made them ill. The company went so far as to blame the women, suggesting that they died of syphilis. Local medical doctors were complicit in the cover up. After protracted legal battle, the Radium Girls settled for damages, medical, and legal expenses. The case is historically significant in the labor movement and workers' right to know.

The publicity created by the Radium Girls ensured that scientists were extremely cautious in handling radioactive material. In 1944, a young chemist was working with plutonium at a secret government laboratory in Los Alamos, New Mexico, when the entire laboratory supply burst open splattering against the wall and into his mouth. He immediately went to the health director's office to have his stomach pumped. Little was known about the effects of plutonium ingestion and the lab assistant monitored his own excretions for plutonium. From this incident, the health director, Louis Hempelmann, expressed concerns regarding the need for studies in the detection of plutonium in bodily secretions. Over the next several months, further concerns were raised that Los Alamos laboratory workers may be overexposed to plutonium. Hempelmann, J. Robert Oppenheimer (the laboratory director), Colonel Robert Stone (the medical director of the Manhattan Project), and other government scientists agreed to conduct "human tracer experiments" to explore excretion. The experiments did not include the Los Alamos staff who were the actual subjects of interest. The experiments proposed injecting one to ten micrograms of plutonium into terminally ill hospital patients and collecting urine and feces to determine excretion rates. The doctor-researchers believed that plutonium had no short-term risks to human health and if the study team selected patients who were expected to die soon, they did not have to worry about long-term effects.

Four sites were selected for the study, Oak Ridge Army Hospital in Tennessee, University of Rochester in New York, University of Chicago, and University of California. Over the course of the study, 18 patients were injected. The first patient was construction worker Ebb Cade. On March 24, 1945, Cade was in an automobile crash and admitted to Oak Ridge Hospital. The 53-year-old African American male suffered fractures of the arm and leg and was otherwise in good health (not at all terminally ill). On April 10, army doctors injected 4.7 micrograms of plutonium into Mr. Cade. Over the next several days, they collected urine, feces, teeth, and bone samples. Data collection ended when Mr. Cade left the hospital without notice. He was later assigned participant number "HP-12." HP was code name for "Human Product." There is no evidence to suggest that Mr. Cade knew that he was injected with radioactive material or that he was in a study tracing radioactive material in his body. At Billings Hospital, University of Chicago, three patients were injected with plutonium. Two of the patients received approximately 95 micrograms of plutonium. The Chicago patients were told that they were being injected with radioactive material. They were not informed of the health risks of the material. All three subsequently died of their primary diagnosis. At the University of Rochester, doctors disregarded the criteria that patients must be terminally ill and specifically chose 11 patients whom they thought would benefit from longer time in the hospital. Six patients were injected with increasingly higher doses of uranium until kidney damage occurred. Five patients were injected with polonium. The patients were never told that they had been injected and the doctors decided it was best not to add a notation in the patient chart. At the University of California, doctors selected two adults and one child for plutonium injection, a teenage male for americium injection and a 55-year-old female cancer patient for zirconium injection. The first California patient was Albert Stevens, a 58-year-old male diagnosed with advanced stomach cancer. Soon after the plutonium injection, gastric biopsy revealed that Stevens had a benign gastric ulcer, not stomach cancer. In addition to bodily excretions, the researchers collected bone and spleen specimens from Mr. Stephens. When Stephens considered moving, the researchers paid him a monthly stipend of $50 to remain in the area. The second California patient was four-year-old Simeon Shaw of Australia. Shaw suffered from osteogenic sarcoma. The Red Cross and U.S. Army flew the young boy and his mother to San Francisco where they believed he would get the best medical care. Within days of arriving, Simeon was injected with plutonium, yttrium, and cerium. Simeon was discharged in May 1946 and died the following January. Hospital notes report that doctors took a bone sample to determine the rate of uptake of radioactive material suggesting that they specifically chose Simeon because of his osteosarcoma.

Children were also used as guinea pigs at the Walter E. Fernald School in Massachusetts. Like many state institutions of the 1940s, Fernald School was crowded, poorly resourced, dirty, and short staffed. Children at the school were from poor families struggling to survive. In 1946, Massachusetts Institute of Technology researchers sought to study the absorption of radioactive iron, calcium, and other minerals in the body. The National Institutes of Health, the Atomic Energy Commission, and Quaker Oats Company funded a study to give children oatmeal laced with radioactive material. One study exposed 17 youth to radioactive iodine. A second study exposed 57 children to radioactive calcium over several years. The scientists recruited teenagers in the science club by promising a special breakfast meal containing calcium, an extra quart of milk, and trips to a baseball game, beach, or restaurant. The medical director and school superintendent, both medical doctors, told parents that the purpose of the study was to improve nutritional status and to "help them." Parents were not informed of the use of radioactive substances or that radioactive substances could be harmful to the child. Mr. Fred Boyce, one of the study subjects later recalled:

> I won't tell you now about the severe physical and mental abuse, but I can assure you, it was no Boys' Town. The idea of getting consent for experiments under these conditions was not only cruel but hypocritical. They bribed us by offering us special privileges, knowing that we had so little that we would do practically anything for attention; and to say, I quote, "This is their debt to society," end quote, as if we were worth no more than laboratory mice, is unforgiveable. (*Advisory Committee on Human Radiation Experiments: Final Report* 1995, Chapter 7)

Boys in the science club were given cereal with radioactive milk for breakfast. Study notes report that three youth objected and researchers "induced" them to change their minds. Investigators later commented that the children were used as guinea pigs because of their vulnerable social position. Promises of milk, oatmeal, or trips to the beach would not have worked for children of wealthier families. Fernald was not the only location of such studies. In 1961, Harvard and Boston University medical researchers administered radioactive iodine to 70 children at Wrentham State School to assess effectiveness of countermeasures to nuclear fallout.

From 1944 to 1974, scientists conducted approximately 4,000 experiments to test the effects of various doses of radiation on humans. Several thousand studies were paid for by the federal government. Among the human radiation studies were:

- The Vanderbilt "Nutrition Study" where 820 poor pregnant women were given radioactive iron to study the absorption of iron during pregnancy.

- Dr. Carl Heller's Oregon State Prison Study where 67 inmates were exposed to the equivalent of 2,400 chest x-rays followed by urine specimens, testicular biopsy, and vasectomy. The men were paid $25 for each testicular biopsy and $25 for the vasectomy. They were also told that participation in the study could influence their parole status.

- The Green Run, one of several intentional releases of radiation into the environment in order to test weapons, safety equipment, or dispersion.

On January 15, 1994, President Bill Clinton appointed the Advisory Committee on Human Radiation Experiments to investigate unethical nuclear experiments funded by the federal government. In the 900-page report, the investigators describe many programs that were conducted in private as researchers hoped to avoid embarrassment, legal liability, and public distrust in government programs. Many of the programs failed to maintain adequate study records or provide informed consent. Study subjects did not realize that they were part of an experiment. In October 1995, Clinton officially apologized to the surviving individuals and their family members for harms caused by the human radiation experiments. The president called for truth and accountability in government-sponsored research.

Research aims to build a body of knowledge. In health and medicine, the body of knowledge is primarily compiled by studying, interacting with, and exploring human experiences, functions, and thoughts. Having a clear vision of the study sample and adhering to the proposed sampling protocol ensures safety of the people who volunteer their time for research as well as use and generalizability of the study results. When study participants overrepresent or misrepresent one gender, ethnic group, or socio-demographic population, faulty conclusions may result. In public health and medicine, nonrepresentative samples can lead to

increased morbidity and mortality of certain minority groups. It is also impera-
tive that researchers honor and respect study participants as human beings with
the right to informed consent. Without study participants, research in health and
psychology could not occur.

FURTHER READING

Advisory Committee on Human Radiation Experiments: Final Report. 1995. Wash-
     ington, D.C.: The Committee: Supt. of Docs., U.S. G.P.O., distributor,
     1995. Accessed June 1, 2018. https://bioethicsarchive.georgetown.edu
     /achre/final/report.html
Atomic Heritage Foundation. 2017. "Human Radiation Experiments." July 11.
     Accessed August 21, 2019. https://www.atomicheritage.org/history
     /human-radiation-experiments
Bardi, Anat, Kathryn E. Buchanan, Robin Goodwin, Letitia Slabu, and Mark Rob-
     inson. 2014. "Value Stability and Change during Self-Chosen Life Transi-
     tions: Self-Selection versus Socialization Effects." *Journal of Personality
     and Social Psychology* 106 (1): 131–47.
Beck, Hall P., Sharman Levinson, and Gary Irons. 2009. "Finding Little Albert:
     A Journey to John B Watson's Infant Laboratory." *American Psycholo-
     gist* 64 (7): 605–14.
Charles, Anna, Annette Rid, Hugh Davies, and Heather Draper. 2016. "Prisoners
     as Research Participants: Current Practice and Attitudes in the UK."
     Journal of Medical Ethics: The Journal of the Institute of Medical Ethics
     42 (4): 246–52.
Cohen, Jodi S. 2018a. "$3 Million Research Breakdown at UIC, Where a Star
     Psychiatrist Put Kids at Risk." *Chicago Sun-Times (IL)*, April 26. *News-
     Bank*, Cohen ProPublica, Illinois. Accessed April 27, 2019. https://www
     .propublica.org/article/university-of-illinois-chicago-mani-pavuluri
     -3-million-research-breakdown
Cohen, Jodi S. 2018b. "Illinois Regulators are Investigating a Psychiatrist Whose
     Research with Children was Marred by Misconduct." *Chronicle of
     Higher Education*, December 12. Accessed December 16, 2019. https://
     www.chronicle.com/article/Illinois-Regulators-Are/245301
Digdon, Nancy. 2017. "The Little Albert Controversy: Intuition, Confirmation
     Bias, and Logic." *History of Psychology* (January 26): 1–10. Advance
     online publication. http://dx.doi.org/10.1037/hop0000055
Fisher, B., and C. K. Redmond. 1994. "Fraud in Breast-Cancer Trials." *The New
     England Journal of Medicine* 330 (20): 1458–62.
Guinea Pig Zero. 2019. Accessed August 28, 2019. https://www.guineapigzero
     .com/

Haggbloom, Steven J., Renee Warnick, Jason E. Warnick, Vinessa K. Jones, Gary
    L. Yarbrough, Tenea M. Russell, Chris M. Borecky, et al. 2002. "The 100
    Most Eminent Psychologists of the 20th Century." *Review of General
    Psychology* 6 (2): 139–52.

Hanel, Paul H. P., and Katia C. Vione. 2016. "Do Student Samples Provide an
    Accurate Estimate of the General Public?" *PLoS ONE* 11 (12): 1–10.

Hornblum, Allen M. 1998. *Acres of Skin: Human Experiments at Holmesburg
    Prison: A Story of Abuse and Exploitation in the Name of Medical Sci-
    ence.* New York: Routledge.

Office of Research Integrity, U.S. Public Health Service. 1993. *ORI Newsletter.*
    April. vol. 1 (2). Accessed August 28, 2019. https://ori.hhs.gov/images
    /ddblock/vol1_no2.pdf

Peterson, Robert A. 2001. "On the Use of College Students in Social Science
    Research: Insights from a Second-Order Meta-Analysis." *Journal of
    Consumer Research* 28 (3): 450–61.

Portenoy, Russell K., and Kathleen M. Foley. 1986. "Chronic Use of Opioid
    Analgesics in Non-Malignant Pain: Report of 38 Cases." *Pain* 25 (2):
    171–86.

Reiter, Keramet. "Experimentation on Prisoners: Persistent Dilemmas in Rights
    and Regulations." *California Law Review* 97 (2) (April 2009): 501–66.

Schroeder, Doris, Julie Cook, François Hirsch, Solveig Fenet, and Vasantha
    Muthuswamy, eds. 2017. "Ethics Dumping: Case Studies from North-
    South Research." Springer Open. Accessed May 5, 2019. https://link
    .springer.com/content/pdf/10.1007%2F978-3-319-64731-9.pdf

U.S. Department of Health and Human Services. 2018. "Youth Risk Behavior
    Surveillance- United States, 2017. *Morbidity and Mortality Weekly
    Reports* 67 (8) (June 15). Accessed January 24, 2018. https://www.cdc
    .gov/healthyyouth/data/yrbs/pdf/2017/ss6708.pdf

Watson, J. B., and R. Rayner. 1920. "Conditioned Emotional Reactions." *Journal
    of Experimental Psychology* 3 (1): 1–14.

SIX

Study Instruments and Data Collection

Data collection is the stage of research where the scientist gathers facts, measurements, or information from the study sample and records observations in the laboratory notebook. The logistics of data collection—how, when, and where data collection will occur—is identified and documented before a study starts. To collect data, the researcher must first decide what variables are relevant to the study and the best way to measure those variables. Items to consider are the purpose of the study, human participant protections, how other researchers measure the variable of interest, available tools, and research budget. The purpose of the study indicates whether the study is quantitative (tests a hypothesis) or qualitative (explores experiences, ideas, or perceptions in order to develop a hypothesis for later study). Quantitative data are numerical and measurable. Qualitative data are thoughts, ideas, stories, images, or other descriptive information. The tool that the researcher uses to gather the data is an *instrument*. The instrument could be a measuring device, survey, or the researcher asking questions. While it is best to use the most accurate tool to gather data, this may not be possible if the tool is very expensive or collecting data is potentially harmful to study participants. To determine the best possible tool for data collection, researchers refer back to the literature. In reviewing past studies, scientists learn what instruments other researchers use to measure the variables of interest and which instrument is the best match for the purpose, needs, and requirements of the proposed study. Once the researcher determines how data will be collected and the independent review board for human participant protections approves the study, the researcher may commence data collection. Although data collection procedures are outlined in advance, the researcher may take further notes during data collection. Clear, concise, and accurate descriptions of data collection procedures are important so that other researchers are able to replicate the procedures. The ability to repeat a study by independent researchers is important in validating study findings and building the discipline's body of knowledge. As with other stages of the scientific method, data collection is vulnerable to errors and misconduct. There are also natural limitations to data collection as researchers push the boundaries of science and research.

Data is the plural form of *datum*. Data are the information collected in order to test a research hypothesis or research question. Raw data are the information collected directly from the study sample without any editing, analysis, or adjustment. Data collection takes a variety of forms depending on the variable, the source of the data, and the purpose of the study. There are often different ways to measure the same variable. For example, in studying bullying in schools, the researcher could look at school records of serious incident reports related to bullying, surveys of student experiences of bullying, teacher or administrator surveys, school nurse records, or direct observations in places where bullying is likely to occur. Each form of data collection has advantages and disadvantages. In a survey of bullying, the respondent may not recognize some behaviors as bullying. As a result, bullying would be underreported. Alternatively, the respondent may attribute malicious intent to actions when there is none, which would result in overreporting. There is no perfect form of data collection. One way to compensate for the limitations of various instruments is to use triangulation. With triangulation, the researcher collects data from multiple sources or by different techniques. Triangulation may be thought of as taking a photo of an object from various angles. Each angle provides a different perspective giving the observer a more comprehensive image than one angle alone.

The study instrument is the device that the researcher uses to measure the variable of interest. If a study investigates the effects of an experimental drug on blood pressure, the most likely instrument is a sphygmomanometer. If a study examines differences in brain activity, the researcher might use positron emission tomography (PET) scan. If a study examines physical activity, the researcher may use an activity monitor. In face-to-face interviews, the person asking the question is the instrument. The actual questions asked are important but not as important as who asks the question. For example, imagine that you took an exam and found it extremely difficult. The test questions were confusing, and you do not think the questions covered the course material. You left feeling dejected and unprepared, even a little angry. As you leave, the instructor asks, "How was the exam?" You politely respond, "OK," or "It was challenging." When you get home, your best friend asks, "How was the exam?" Both the instructor and your friend asked the same question. The answer to your friend is probably quite different. Answers vary based on who is asking the question. For this reason, in individual or group interviews, the person asking the question is the instrument.

The study instrument is determined during the planning stage of the study. The researcher can either use an instrument that already exists or develop a new instrument. If an instrument exists and the cost is not prohibitive, it makes sense to use the same instrument that other scientists use. Using the same instrument allows the researcher to make comparisons between current study results and other researchers' results. In some cases, the researcher may opt to develop a new instrument. Instrument development is actually a novel research study in and of itself. To develop a new survey, the researcher must state each question clearly so that the reader can understand and answer the question correctly. After development, the researcher pilot tests the instrument and validates the instrument against other instruments. The quality of a research instrument is assessed by reliability and validity. Reliability assesses the consistency or stability of the instrument. For example, a metal ruler is a reliable instrument to measure height. The ruler will accurately measure the same height of a person at different points in time provided the person does not grow taller or lose height. Under the same circumstances, the ruler will yield the same measurement. Validity describes how well the instrument measures what it is intended to measure. A ruler is a valid instrument to measure length. It is less valid in measuring weight, volume (without complex calculations), or age. There are different types of validity. Face validity assesses whether the instrument seems to be a reasonable measure of the variable of interest. Criterion validity is the degree to which the instrument relates to some external scale measuring a related variable. Content validity assesses how well the instrument covers the range of meanings within the variable of interest. Construct validity assesses how well the instrument reflects the theoretical concepts of the variable of interest. The terms *reliability* and *validity* of an instrument can be confusing because they are also used to assess the overall quality of the study.

Good record-keeping is critical to scientific discovery and hypothesis testing. Failure to maintain clear documentation of study results can lead to confusion or skepticism over results. Yet many scientists are not formally trained in how to document study methods. Best practices in scientific record-keeping suggest:

- Keeping a dedicated laboratory notebook, either a written or electronic notebook.
- Recording all raw data immediately after collection (rather than writing on scrap paper and then transferring the data into the notebook).
- Noting the date and time of each data collection.
- Writing clearly and legibly in ink.
- Documenting any edits with date, time, and reason for the edit.
- Regular review and approval by the supervisor or other responsible party.

- Clear description of study methods, instrument calibrations, thoughts, and impressions related to data collection.

- Storing all data in a secure location to ensure human participant protections.

- Maintaining a backup of all electronic records with password protection.

- Saving any photographs, recordings, hard copies of instruments, or meeting notes in a second notebook or file folder.

The laboratory notebook is an invaluable tool. It is a notebook, a journal of professional activity, and a place to record important insights, whether the insights occur during data collection or not. The recorded comments and notes may be helpful in planning future studies.

Ideally, the stage of data collection will go smoothly, just as the scientist planned, results will be neat and clear, and the researcher can prove the hypothesis. Unfortunately, that is not how things usually go. There are limitations to instrumentation, unexpected events, surprising results, and not all discoveries occur during data collection. Discoveries may occur out of order.

LIMITATIONS ON MEASUREMENT

A major limitation of data collection is that scientists can only measure variables that we have instruments to measure. For example, the well-known sex researcher, Alfred Kinsey was criticized for measuring sexual interactions based on biology and overlooking the psychological aspect of sexuality. Despite his controversial methods, Kinsey opened a new line of research that later yielded better ways to measure sexual response. Finding or developing a valid and reliable instrument can be very challenging. Consider body mass index (BMI) as an example. BMI is a common way to measure or define body composition, whether someone is underweight, normal weight, overweight, or obese. Despite overwhelming use, BMI has limitations. BMI estimates body fat based on height and weight. Because muscle is denser than fat, athletes and bodybuilders often fall within the overweight or obese range. This means that BMI is not a good instrument for athletes. There are other ways to measure body composition. However, some require expensive equipment, a major obstacle for small studies. In other research, studies have investigated how well students learn when they listen to music or how well students do on standardized tests when they chew gum. The challenge for the researcher is how to accurately measure learning or test taking. In general, there is no perfect instrument. Scientists aim to measure the variable of interest in the most accurate way possible within the constraints of time, resources, and available instruments.

Sensitivity and specificity assess the quality of a clinical test and the test's cutoff values. Cutoff values are the points of a test result where above or equal to that value is considered positive while below the value is considered negative. The cutoff value of obesity by BMI is 30.0 or higher. Sensitivity is the ability of a test to accurately identify people with disease as having the disease (true positives). Specificity is the ability of a test to correctly identify people without disease as not having the disease (true negatives). There is a tradeoff between sensitivity and specificity. High sensitivity increases the chance of false positives, people who do not have disease but screen positive. Mammograms are an example of a test with high sensitivity. Mammograms correctly identify about 87 percent of women with breast cancer (Lehman et al. 2017). However, in increasing sensitivity, false positives also increase. After 10 years of annual mammograms, about half of women will have at least one false positive result (Hubbard et al. 2011). While the false positive mammogram would later be ruled out with subsequent testing, the initial result creates unnecessary anxiety. The number of false negatives, people who screen negative for a disease but are actually positive, increases with high specificity. The blood test for prostate cancer, prostate-specific antigen (PSA) test, has 93 percent specificity. However, 15–38 percent of men with cancer have PSA levels within normal limits. Experts who determine the cutoff values for PSA point out that few men die of prostate cancer. Lowering specificity may not impact mortality rates for prostate cancer. Determining the cutoff values of a particular laboratory test is a balancing act between sensitivity and specificity.

ADVERSE EVENTS

During the course of an experiment, some treatments may cause undesirable side effects. For example, a clinical trial of a chemotherapeutic agent among patients with cancer will very likely increase risk of opportunistic infection. Study participants are advised of this risk in the informed consent process. Adverse events refer to *unexpected* symptoms, abnormal laboratory findings, disease, or injury experienced by a study participant during a research study or associated by time with a study. Definition varies by research discipline. For example, the National Cancer Institute definition focuses on clinical trials of chemotherapy drugs and specifically defines adverse events as previously unknown toxicities or life-threatening toxicities, regardless of whether the problem was previously known or suspected. The Common Rule (see chapter 2) does not specifically use the term *adverse event* and instead uses the term *unanticipated problems*. In general, any undesirable experience of a study participant related to the experimental use of medical technology, pharmaceutical agent, or behavioral intervention may be considered an adverse event. Adverse events that create disability, birth defect, life-threatening reaction, or require inpatient hospitalization or prolongation of current hospitalization are classified as *serious adverse events*. In the case of Dan Markingson and the CAFE study (chapter 2), Markingson's marked behavioral changes of grandiosity and delusions would be classified as an adverse event. His death due to suicide was classified as a severe adverse event. The primary investigator is responsible for reporting any adverse events to the IRB as well as any relevant data safety monitoring board or funding organization. The IRB determines whether the study should be suspended or terminated. Adverse events, when a healthy study volunteer suddenly becomes ill or dies, is one of the most horrifying events in research.

Jesse Gelsinger

Jesse Gelsinger was born with the rare genetic disorder Ornithine transcarbamylase (OTC) deficiency. OTC deficiency allows a byproduct of protein breakdown, ammonia, to accumulate in the blood. Increased ammonia levels damage the nervous system. Symptoms of hyperammonemia include vomiting, tiredness, personality changes, confusion, seizures, and coma and may lead to death. The X-linked disorder affects between 1 in 14,000 and 1 in 77,000 people. Approximately half of all infants born with OTC deficiency die within the first month, many within the first 72 hours of birth. Jesse had partial OTC deficiency. His disorder went undetected during infancy because Jesse was breastfed. As a toddler, Jesse refused to eat meat or dairy products. By age two and a half, his parents noticed their son appeared lethargic and belligerent. Jesse's doctor suggested a high protein diet. Within days of the new diet, Jesse went into a coma. His parents took him the Children's Hospital of Philadelphia where he was diagnosed with OTC deficiency. Throughout his childhood, Jesse occasionally tested the limits of his disease. Illness and hospitalization quickly turned him back to his regimen of a strict low protein diet and about 50 pills a day. Like many teenagers with chronic illness, Jesse rebelled against his disease. When he learned of a Phase I clinical trial that could help save newborns with OTC deficiency, he was eager to volunteer. He waited patiently for his 18th birthday so that he could participate in the study. On his 18th birthday, Jesse and his family flew from their home in Arizona to Philadelphia. At the University of Pennsylvania Institute for Human Gene Therapy, Jesse was screened for the study. His blood ammonia level was 47 µ/dl, only slightly above normal blood-ammonia levels of 15–45 µ/dl. The protocol excluded study participants with blood-ammonia levels above 75 µ/dl. Jesse and his family flew home with plans for Jesse to return when it was his turn for the study procedure. When one study volunteer dropped out of the study, Jesse's chance came earlier than expected.

Gene therapy works by replacing the dysfunctional gene with functional genes. Weakened viruses serve as vectors carrying the corrective DNA fragments into the cell nucleus. The typical vector is a cold virus. From the start, Jesse knew that he would not benefit from the gene therapy. His body would attack any cells carrying the virus and, in the process, destroy the corrective gene. Jesse still wanted to be part of the study. He wanted to help infants with OTC deficiency and other genetic disorders. On September 12, 1999, Jesse returned to Philadelphia for the gene therapy experiment. The co-investigators of the trial were Dr. Mark Batshaw, a pediatrician, and Dr. James Wilson, an expert in gene therapy. On arrival, Jesse's ammonia level was 91 μ/dl. His doctors decided to proceed with the study. On September 13, the doctor-researcher administered drugs to reduce Jesse's blood ammonia level and injected the infusion of the corrective *OTC* gene encased in a cold virus into his hepatic vein. Jesse received the highest dose of the adenovirus vector-corrective gene treatment given to any study participant. Within 18 hours, Jesse developed severe jaundice. His body rapidly deteriorated and he progressed to multi-system organ failure. His ammonia levels peaked to 393 μ/dl. Within four days of the experimental infusion, the rebellious, heroic, and seemingly invincible teenager was brain dead and his body was relieved of life support machinery.

Doctors later determined that Jesse experienced a severe allergic reaction to the cold virus. The study team had expected some reaction to the vector. Several previous study participants had experienced side effects. The adenovirus would most likely cause fever or cold-like symptoms. During animal trials, three rhesus monkeys died of a clotting disorder from a stronger version of the vector. Several monkeys suffered severe liver failure after receiving the same vector as Jesse. On October 11, the FDA suspended the Batshaw-Wilson study, banning any new study participants. Current participants were allowed to complete the study. The adenovirus vector that Jesse received was currently being used in about 50 gene therapy trials. On November 3, the *Washington Post* reported six deaths in gene therapy experiments. The cases were not reported to the FDA. Public hearings of the Gelsinger case were held on November 9–10. Subsequent investigation revealed failure by the co-investigators to inform study participants of the animal deaths and illnesses, failure to report that two other study participants had suffered reactions at lower doses, changing the order of study participants without seeking prior approval from the IRB, and proceeding with Jesse's injection despite high blood ammonia levels. On January 21, 2000, the FDA shut down all gene therapy studies at University of Pennsylvania citing numerous deficiencies. In late January, a second research lab suspended their gene therapy experiment after three of the six patients died and a seventh became seriously ill. The FDA was flooded with reports of adverse events in gene therapy trials. Six hundred and ninety-one volunteers had become ill or died in the seven years prior to Jesse's death. Only three of the adverse events were reported to the FDA. The investigation also revealed that Wilson was a major shareholder in the company funding the Institute for Human Gene Therapy. If the adenovirus vector had been successful in inserting the gene fragments, the vector could be used to treat other genetic disorders. The gene therapy treatment would have made shareholders very wealthy. Concerned with the lack of reporting, loose oversight, and potential for conflict of interest, the FDA implemented the Gene Therapy Clinical Trial Monitoring Plan and the Gene Transfer Safety Symposia. The monitoring plan requires clinical monitoring before a trial begins and study team members cannot hold stock in the company sponsoring the trial.

Merck and Vioxx

In 1999, Merck & Co. launched the Vioxx Gastrointestinal Outcomes Research (VIGOR) study to compare their nonsteroidal, anti-inflammatory product Vioxx to an older anti-inflammatory drug naproxen. Eight thousand and seventy-six study participants with rheumatoid arthritis were randomly assigned to treatment groups. Initial results showed that Vioxx had fewer cases of ulcers and gastrointestinal bleeding than naproxen. A month later, the VIGOR safety panel reviewed data showing that serious heart problems and deaths were twice as high in the group taking Vioxx. The data and safety monitoring board voted to continue the study with an amended plan to monitor cardiovascular events among study participants. Panel members thought that naproxen may have been acting as a protection against heart disease, similar to baby aspirin. At the suggestion of the board, Merck reluctantly agreed to analyze the data on heart problems in February 2000. On February 7, the chair of the safety monitoring board reported $72,975 in Merck stock. A month later, the chair signed a contract to consult with Merck for the rate of $5,000 per day. In May, Merck submitted the VIGOR study to the *New England Journal of Medicine* (*NEJM*) for peer review. The article only included 17 of the 20 heart attacks among Vioxx patients. Merck reported the heart attacks to the FDA in October. The article, published in the *NEJM* in November still failed to mention the actual number of adverse cardiac events. Repeated analyses of the VIGOR study data by external reviewers showed higher risk of heart attack among Vioxx users. By the time Vioxx was taken off the market, experts estimated that 20 million Americans had taken Vioxx, 88,000 suffered from heart attack while on Vioxx, and 38,000 patients died from heart attacks (Prakash and Valentine 2007). In November 2007, Merck announced the legal settlement of $4.85 billion. The settlement allowed the pharmaceutical company to avoid approximately 47,000 personal-injury lawsuits.

DEFYING NATURE

The early science-fiction novel *Frankenstein* by Mary Shelley is the classic story of experimentation gone awry. Shelley's writing was based on research by Luigi Galvani and his nephew, Giovanni Aldini. Galvani experimented with electricity to stimulate the leg muscle of dead frogs. Aldini took his uncle's experiments to the next level, experimenting on the body of a recently executed criminal. Although Galvani and Aldini (thankfully) failed in their mission, the potential for developing or exposing the general public to hazardous materials through experimentation does exist. There have been several incidents of laboratory monkeys escaping or being intentionally released from research laboratories by animal rights activists. In 1991, 82 monkeys escaped from New Mexico State University AIDS research center after their cages were knocked over by high winds. All monkeys were recovered and did not pose a danger to the public. In a 1989 case, scientists discovered a new strain of the deadly Ebola virus in laboratory monkeys at Hazleton Laboratories in Reston, Virginia. The discovery raised quite a scare because of the proximity of Reston to the Washington, D.C. metropolitan area. The lab tested all of their animal handlers. Six of 178 laboratory technicians tested positive for the Reston virus. Although the strain was lethal to some monkeys, it did not cause illness in humans. There have also been cases of intentional harm by scientists. In September 2001, letters containing anthrax were sent to NBC News, the *New York Post*, and two democratic senators. Twenty-two people were infected. Five people died. The FBI traced the anthrax strain to the U.S. Army Medical Research Institute of Infectious Diseases, Fort Detrick, Maryland, and microbiologist Bruce Edwards Ivins. Ivins died by suicide before he was charged with any crime. Investigators believe that Ivins was using the attacks to salvage funding for his research project finding a vaccine against anthrax.

In manipulating nature, scientists raise the possibility of intentional or unintentional manmade disasters. Gain-of-function (GOF) studies are one area of great scientific concern. GOF experiments strengthen a pathogen's ability to cause disease. Advocates claim that GOF studies help infectious disease and public health specialists understand viruses and how epidemics spread. Critics raise concerns that the manipulated pathogen could escape and create a pandemic. In 2011, virologist Ron Fouchier of Erasmus Medical Center in The Netherlands and Yoshihiro Kawaoka of University of Wisconsin–Madison separately announced that they had created a particularly virulent strain of H5N1 avian influenza virus. The strain was more powerful than anthrax. As with other scientific studies, the scientists wanted to publish their studies. The study methods would have essentially provided instructions for bioterrorists on how to create a lethal weapon. After review by the U.S. National Science Advisory Board for Biosecurity and much public debate, the studies were eventually published. In 2014, the Fouchier and Kawaoka research teams and other GOF researchers agreed to a temporary moratorium on research. Experiments resumed in 2013 and were paused again after three incidents of poor laboratory practices at the U.S. Centers for Disease Control and Prevention (CDC) (Kaiser 2014). In the first incident, six vials of smallpox stored at the National Institutes of Health in Bethesda, Maryland, tested positive for live virus. The virus was thought to be dead and unable to cause an outbreak. In a second incident, 75 CDC staff were exposed to live anthrax that was also thought to be dead. In the third incident, the CDC staff sent what they thought was a sample of low-pathogenic H9N2 avian influenza to a U.S. Department of Agriculture (USDA) lab only to find out the sample contained a highly virulent strain of H5N1 avian influenza. Studies resumed in 2019 under a new set of guidelines requiring careful consideration and oversight of risk vs. benefit. The case of Africanized honeybees demonstrates the ease of unintentional release of hazardous samples into a community and the consequences.

Killer Bees

In 1956, the Brazilian Ministry of Agriculture asked environmentalist Warwick Estevam Kerr to create a hybrid honeybee that would increase Brazilian honey production. Kerr traveled to Africa where he retrieved samples of Tanzanian honeybee queens. The African honeybee is extraordinarily industrious, working early in the day and late into the evening. Unlike traditional European bees, the African honeybee continues to gather nectar in cool weather. The plan was to crossbreed African honeybees with the European strains to increase honey production in Brazil. Kerr imported 90 fertilized queens. Each queen was kept in a separate hive at a quarantine station in southeastern Brazil. Each hive contained a mesh screen to prevent the queen from escaping. A guard watched over the hives. One Sunday, when the guard was off duty, a local beekeeper visited. He thought that the excluder screens were blocking honey production and removed them. Kerr did not realize what had happened for almost three weeks. Twenty-six Tanzanian queen bees swarmed the hive. Swarming is a behavior where the queen and thousands of worker and drone bees leave the original hive to start a new hive. Each queen takes about 20,000–30,000 workers and drones with her. Before the bees swarm, they consume a lot of honey. European honeybees will normally swarm once or twice a year. A new queen and worker and drone bees are left to maintain the original hive. Kerr reported the escape to the Department of Agriculture. They assumed the aggressive genetics would be diluted by continued cross-breeding with native bees. They quickly learned that the aggressiveness of African bees is not limited to honey production. The African bee angers easily, attacks people and animals without provocation, and swarms three or more times a year. The Africanized bee swarms took over the hives of European and South American bees, killing the queen and replacing her with a new queen. Within three years, locals reported bee attacks on chicken and pigs. In 1963, Africanized bees attacked and killed the first human. The bees are known to chase victims a quarter of a mile and are currently taking over the habitat of native honeybees in the southern United States. Kerr felt responsible for the outbreak. He spent the rest of his life studying ways to manage the hybrid bees.

CONFIRMATION BIAS

Scientists must commit a great deal of time, effort, and resources to their research. When the FBI investigated Bruce Edwards Ivins as the source of the 2001 anthrax attacks, they found that he had spent nearly 30 years of his life working on treatments and vaccines for anthrax. He was so highly invested in his research that he overlooked the moral and social implications of infecting people with anthrax. In order to invest time and effort into researching a particular problem, the scientist must have some degree of emotional investment in the topic. Such personal dedication is a good quality, unless it interferes with the scientist's ability to act as a neutral observer (or facilitates bioterrorism). Pathological science (described in chapter 1) is unintentional self-delusion by scientists where existing beliefs influence experimental observations and data collection. Confirmation bias is the tendency to seek, interpret, or record results that support existing beliefs or theory. Pathological science and confirmation bias are very similar. The main difference is that confirmation bias extends beyond scientific experimentation and can apply to everyday life. With confirmation bias, the person avoids ideas that challenge current modes of thinking and prefers information that reinforces current beliefs. Conspiracy theories are a good example of confirmation bias. Conspiracy theorists seek out information that supports the conspiracy while rejecting information that refutes the conspiracy. In terms of data collection, confirmation bias may cause a scientist to interpret a threshold value in favor of the research hypothesis or to toss out values that do not support the preferred hypothesis. When the scientist intentionally changes or omits data to support a hypothesis, the action is data falsification, a form of research misconduct. Data falsification is discussed in chapter 7. Clever Hans is a well-known example of confirmation bias in psychology.

Clever Hans

Clever Hans was a horse owned by Wilhelm von Osten in the early 1900s. Von Osten lived in Berlin, Germany. The retired math teacher spent many hours teaching his horse math, reading, music, and other lessons. Von Osten's goal was to prove that animals could think and reason. After several years, Clever Hans could tap out the answer to complex mathematical problems, recognize colors, identify people from old photographs, count the number of windows of nearby buildings, and even identify dissonant chords in classical music. His knowledge was amazing. To communicate his success, von Osten took out a notice in the local newspapers. He offered free demonstrations of animal intelligence. Before long, the demonstrations attracted numerous people including some very famous people. Zoologists, high-ranking military officials, equestrians, and psychologists observed and confirmed the horse's incredible cognitive abilities. Stories of Clever Hans regularly appeared in newspapers and magazines. He was featured on postcards and liquor bottle labels. The demonstration also raised serious philosophical questions. If man was superior to animals, how could this animal answer questions that some humans could not answer? As debate over Clever Hans grew, von Osten invited educated scholars to observe the horse and to confirm animal intelligence. The Hans Commission was created consisting of a circus manager, a teacher, the Director of the Berlin Zoological Garden, and the chair of the Department of Sense-Physiology at the University of Berlin. The group carefully observed von Osten, Clever Hans, and people in the audience who could be secretly signaling the horse. The horse tapped out answers to questions with almost 100 percent accuracy. The Hans Commission concluded that they could not detect any signals or trickery by Osten or members of the audience. The crowds flocked to the small square by von Osten's home to see the curious phenomenon.

Oskar Pfungst, a graduate student at the Department of Sense-Physiology, University of Berlin devised a series of experiments to rule out other possible explanations for the animal's uncharacteristic behavior. Pfungst suspected that Clever Hans was reacting to some unintentional signal by the questioner. Pfungst's experiments included a series of tests where Clever Hans was shown a number written on a card. When the person asking the questions could see the number, Clever Hans tapped out the correct answer 98 percent of the time. When the questioner could not see the number, Clever Hans tapped out the correct answer only 8 percent of the time. For the next experiment, Pfungst placed blinders on the horse. The horse aggressively twisted and turned to see the person asking the questions. When the horse was able to twist into a position where he could see the person, he tapped out the correct answer 89 percent of the time. When he could not see the questioner, accuracy rate dropped to 6 percent. It was clear that the horse had picked up subtle signals. What was actually happening was that Clever Hans was often hungry. Hans quickly learned that he would get a treat if he tapped his foot while the questioner looked down and stopped tapping when the questioner looked up. The head movement was barely detectable, but enough for the hungry horse. Von Osten was very upset. He expected Pfungst's experiments to support his animal intelligence hypothesis, not refute it. Initially, von Osten came up with all sorts of reasons why Clever Hans made mistakes. That is, Clever Hans was tired. Clever Hans did not like the questioner. Clever Hans did not like certain types of music. In the end, von Osten refused to allow scientists to observe Clever Hans.

Von Osten suffered from confirmation bias. He believed that Clever Hans could think and reason. He overlooked the obvious question of how the horse learned to read, spell, compute, and detect musical compositions faster than the normal human being. Heinzen, Lilienfeld, and Nolan (2015) compare confirmation bias to the Texas sharpshooter fallacy. The fallacy purports that Texas sharpshooters shoot holes in a barn and then draw bull's eyes around the densest clusters of holes. Observers assume that the bull's eye came before the holes and the shooter is a skilled marksman. Confirmation bias gives the impression that the results support the desired hypothesis by selecting which data to report.

EXPERIMENTER BIAS

Experimenter bias is a condition where the scientist influences the study results. Biases can emerge in different ways, such as the choice of study design or study instrument or through interaction with participants. During data collection, the researcher may provide the study participant with verbal or nonverbal cues that direct the study participant toward a desirable response. Also known as the observer-expectancy effect, Clever Hans is an example of experimenter bias. Von Osten and others questioning the horse provided subtle cues for the horse to stop tapping his foot. The Stanford Prison Experiment is a famous case of experimenter bias. In the Stanford Prison Experiment, study participants were concerned that the researcher would not find what he was looking for so they prompted the study along in some very drastic and evil ways.

Stanford Prison Experiment

During the summer of 1971, a small help wanted advertisement appeared in the local Palo Alto newspaper. The ad offered $15 per day to male college students willing to participate in a one- to two-week psychological study of prison life. With minimum hourly wage at $1.60 per hour, the study paid a fair amount for unskilled labor (U.S. Department of Labor n.d.). Over 70 applicants responded to the advertisement. Applicants were told that the study examined the social roles of prisoners and prison guards. The study protocol excluded anyone with pre-existing mental health problems, medical conditions, history of substance abuse, or history of criminality. Twenty-four participants were selected for inclusion. Eighteen participants were randomly assigned to the role of prison guard or prisoner. The remaining volunteers were assigned as alternatives in case a participant dropped out of the study. Without warning, the researchers conspired with local police to pick up the study participants assigned to the role of prisoner. In a mock arrest, actual police officers picked up each participant, advised him of his legal rights, and searched and handcuffed the suspect in public view. The suspects were then taken to the local police station with flashing lights and sirens. Each participant was identified, charged with robbery, booked, fingerprinted, and blindfolded. They were later transferred—still with blindfold—to the basement of Stanford University's Psychology Department. The basement was set up as a prison. Confused, bewildered, and humiliated, each prisoner was greeted by undergraduate student David Jaffe acting in the role of prison warden. Jaffe informed each prisoner of the seriousness of the purported offense. The prisoner was then stripped naked, searched, and sprayed with delousing solution. Personal clothing was replaced with loose dress-like smocks. The prisoner could wear no underwear, effectively depersonalizing the individual and creating a sense of vulnerability. Names were replaced with prison numbers. A stocking cap simulated a shaved head. The prisoner wore a chain attached to one foot for 24 hours a day to remind him of his captivity. The entire experience was designed to create oppression and subjugation.

The research study was the brainchild of Stanford University psychology professor, Dr. Philip Zimbardo. Journalist Gina Perry (2018) describes Zimbardo as flamboyant, dramatic, and seductive, a man who was later elected president of the American Psychological Association and honored with the American Psychological Foundation's gold medal for lifetime achievement. Funded by the U.S. Office of Naval Research, the purpose of the study was to "understand the development of norms and the effects of roles, labels, and social expectations in a simulated prison environment" (Zimbardo 1999–2019). To simulate the prison experience at Stanford, clocks were removed from the walls, inside doors were replaced with steel-reinforced doors, each cell was labeled with a number, and a small closet measuring two feet by two feet became solitary confinement. The lack of clocks or windows combined with sleep-depriving activities distorted the prisoners' sense of time and place. Cameras and audio tapes were set up to record activity and conversations in the cells and hallway. One obstacle to the simulation was that the toilets were down the hall outside of the mock prison area. The only way to maintain the guise was to blindfold and escort the prisoners to the bathroom. Prisoners were chained together and blindfolded with paper bags over their heads for toilet breaks. Study volunteers assigned to the role of guard wore khaki uniforms with reflective aviator sunglasses and carried a truncheon and whistle. Zimbardo reported that the guards received no training other than the instruction to maintain control of the prisoners. Three guards worked in eight-hour shifts supervising nine prisoners. Zimbardo filled the roles of both researcher and prison superintendent.

By the second day of the experiment, the prisoners revolted. They removed their caps and numbers and barricaded the cell doors. The guards called in the off-duty guards as reinforcements and sprayed the prisoners with fire extinguishers to push them back from the doors. The leader of the rebellion was placed in solitary confinement. The incident worried the guards. The guards were outnumbered on each shift. To prevent further insurrection, the guards developed strategies for psychological control. They offered privileges to a select few prisoners and randomly shifted the privileges from one prisoner to another in order to create confusion and distrust. The mind games worked. The prisoners no longer functioned as a cohesive unit. However, the guards continued to worry. They became more aggressive physically and mentally toward the prisoners. Going to the bathroom became a privilege. After 10:00 p.m., the prisoners had to use a bucket if they needed to urinate or defecate. The buckets, cells, and prisoners began to stink. By the third day, Prisoner #8612 showed signs of acute emotional breakdown with uncontrollable crying and anger. The researchers encouraged him to stay in the study, promising to end the harassment in exchange for information on the other prisoners. The offer did not work. Prisoner #8612's breakdown continued and the researchers had to release him from the study.

The fourth day was visiting day for family and friends. The prison area was cleaned up. The prisoners were shaved, permitted to bathe, and given a nice dinner. Music played over the intercom as a former Stanford University cheerleader greeted the visitors. Visits were restricted to two visitors for ten minutes per prisoner. A few parents complained that their son appeared tired or distressed. Zimbardo shifted blame onto the study participant, suggesting that their son was weak. The concerned parents left without further complaint. On visiting day, there was a rumor that Prisoner #8612 was going to come back with friends and break the other prisoners out. The guards responded by chaining the prisoners together, placing bags over their heads and taking them to a storage room on the fifth floor as soon as visiting time ended. The attempted prison break never occurred. However, the guards felt inconvenienced, frustrated, and angry by the unnecessary move. Physical punishment and humiliation escalated. The guards made the prisoners clean the toilets with their hands. The previously used punishment of push-ups or jumping jackets expanded to several hours.

On the fifth day, Zimbardo's girlfriend, Christina Maslach visited the prison to interview the guards and prisoners. A recent doctoral graduate, Maslach had carefully listened to Zimbardo's descriptions and updates on the study. She was horrified by the sight of the young men marched to the toilets in chains with bags over their heads. Zimbardo and Maslach argued. However, Zimbardo took heed and immediately ended the study. Zimbardo (1999–2019) later reported that of approximately 50 people who visited the prison simulation, Maslach was the only one who objected to the events.

The Stanford Prison Experiment is often reported in psychology textbooks as methodologically flawed with heavy biases in participant selection and researcher demands. In advertising for students to participate in a study of prison life, the researchers may have inadvertently attracted more aggressive and less empathetic individuals than if they had simply advertised for participants in a nondescript psychological study (Bartels 2016). Zimbardo's dual roles as prison superintendent and primary investigator influenced the guards' behavior. John Mark, one of the college students randomized to the role of guard later reflected on the study noting, "Zimbardo went out of his way to create tension. . . . I felt that throughout the experiment, he knew what he wanted and then tried to shape the experiment"

(Ratnesar 2011). Dave Eshleman, the guard that the prisoners nicknamed John Wayne for his unusually aggressive behavior, described his role:

> What came over me was not an accident. It was planned. I set out with a definite plan in mind, to try to force the action, force something to happen, so that the researchers would have something to work with . . . I consciously created this persona . . . "How far can I push these things and how much abuse will these people take before they say, 'knock it off?'" But the other guards didn't stop me. They seemed to join in. (Ratnesar 2011)

Critics of the Stanford Prison Experiment claim that Zimbardo instigated the abuse (Haslam, Reicher, and McDermott 2015). Wanting to impress Zimbardo, the guards acted in ways that they might not normally have acted if the professor had not consciously or unconsciously encouraged aggression. In 2002, the British Broadcasting Corporation (BBC) replicated parts of the Stanford Prison Experiment in a documentary. The purpose of the BBC case was to investigate how people identify with their social group, how people challenge existing status within the group, and how leadership emerges over time. The BBC study lasted eight days and included 15 randomly assigned participants. The prison guards in the BBC experiment never resorted to the level of violence seen in the Stanford Prison Experiment. Despite multiple flaws with the research protocol and clear violation of the principle of do no harm, Zimbardo built a career on the Stanford Prison Experiment.

OWNERSHIP OF DATA

Data are intellectual property and as property, they have monetary value. Data ownership refers to the right to access, create, modify, exclude, sell, or derive benefit from study data. In addition to the right to control the use of the data, the data owner is also responsible for protecting the data, particularly if the data involves confidential personal information. Typically, whoever sponsors the research owns the data. If a scientist is working for a pharmaceutical company, the pharmaceutical company has exclusive rights to any intellectual property procured through work in their laboratory. If a scientist works for a university, the university has intellectual property rights. The researcher has stewardship rights and responsibilities. This means that the researcher may publish the results and transfer copyright to a journal publisher. The steward is also responsible for protecting the data from misuse. Ultimately, the university owns the data. If the investigator leaves an institution, it is good practice to keep a copy of the data in case questions arise. Such arrangements must be made in advance with the sponsoring institution.

As the public becomes more aware of the value of data and intellectual property, issues of ownership are likely to emerge. Such was the case of *Moore v. Regents of the University of California.* In 1976, John Moore went to UCLA Medical Center for treatment of hairy cell leukemia. His doctor, Dr. David Golde, determined that Moore's spleen needed to be removed. Golde also realized that Moore's spleen cells could be used to develop a commercial cell line for biomedical research. Before the surgery, Golde discussed the business and scientific opportunities of the spleen cells with Shirley G. Quan, a researcher with the Regents of the University of California. The doctor arranged for Quan to receive samples of Moore's spleen after removal. They did not tell Moore of the plans. Golde created a cell line from Moore's white blood cells. The Regents applied for a patent on the line with Golde and Quan listed as inventors.

After the surgery, Moore moved to Seattle. He was called back to UCLA several times to provide blood, skin, bone marrow, and sperm samples. When he asked if he could have his medical care transferred to a doctor closer to home, Golde offered to pay Moore's travel expenses. In 1983, Moore was presented with a consent form granting the University of California all rights to his cell line. He signed the consent form but later took the document to a lawyer. The attorney discovered the commercial cell line and payments to Golde for the "Mo" cells. Moore sued on the grounds that Golde and the Board of Regents failed to disclose their financial interest in his cells and failed to obtain informed consent for the procedure. The California Supreme Court ruled in favor of the Regents because the tissue samples were considered discarded property and no longer Moore's property. The Regents later settled with Moore. The *Moore v. Regents of the University of California* case is a landmark legal case for patients and family members who sue researchers over the use of bodily fluids or body parts. Discarded fluid samples or biopsies are generally considered the institution's property, not patient property. The case of Henrietta Lacks mirrors the Moore case except Henrietta's cell line was not discovered until years after her death.

Henrietta Lacks

Loretta Pleasant (1920–1951), later known as Henrietta Lacks, was born in Roanoke Virginia to poor tobacco farmers. When "Hennie" was four years old, her mother died in childbirth. Henrietta and her nine siblings were separated and dispersed among relatives. Henrietta was sent to her grandfather's log cabin in Clover, Virginia. She shared a bedroom with her cousin David "Day" Lacks. The children worked the tobacco fields and attended a segregated school. At the age of 14, Henrietta gave birth to her first child, Lawrence. By the age of 20, she gave birth to her second child and married Day, the father of the children. At the urging of a relative, the couple moved to Maryland. Day worked at Bethlehem Steel.

The Lacks had three more children. At the start of the fifth pregnancy, Henrietta told friends about feeling a knot in her lower abdomen. When the knot did not go away after the birth, Henrietta went to Johns Hopkins Hospital. Johns Hopkins was one of the only hospitals in the area that accepted people of color. Henrietta's doctor, Howard W. Jones, took a biopsy of the tumor and diagnosed cancer of the cervix. The cervical cancer was treated with radium tubes. During the treatments, Jones took further samples and sent samples to George Otto Gey, a cancer researcher at Johns Hopkins. Gey needed cancer cells for his research, but he was having trouble keeping the cells alive. Henrietta's cells not only stayed alive outside of her body, they thrived and reproduced! As was the practice of the day, Gey named the cells "HeLa," using the first two initials of the first and last name of the patient. Henrietta died on October 4, 1951, at the age of 31.

Gey shared the cells with other scientists. HeLa cells are used widely in scientific experiments. Jonas Salk used HeLa cells to develop the polio vaccine. In 1964, the cells were sent into space to determine the impact of space travel on human biology. The cells have been used to study sickle cell anemia, salmonella, cervical cancer, HIV, tuberculosis, and Ebola. The cells assisted in three Nobel Prize awards and allowed scientists to develop the HPV vaccine, chemotherapeutic agents, and to map human genomes. While HeLa cells were being given, sold, and traded across the international scientific community, the Lacks family had no idea that part of their mother's body lived on. Their first clue came in 1973 when a scientist tracked down family members and requested blood samples. To learn that a part of their mother had been taken without her consent and was manipulated to produce commercial products and medical advancements was shocking. Even more ironically, many members of the Lacks family could not afford the medical care and treatments that resulted from her cell line. In 2013, the family was further violated when researchers in Germany published the genome sequence of HeLa cells. The sequence was chaotic with numerous regions of surplus or missing genes. The idea was to allow researchers working with the HeLa cell line to identify any contamination. Instead, the publication revealed private health information without the family's consent. The researchers apologized and withdrew the genome information. Lacks family members now serve on an NIH committee to review health, medical, and biomedical research involving the HeLa genome.

SABOTAGE

There is enormous pressure to publish or perish in science. Perceived competition, greed, envy, distress, and lack of internal moral control can lead to lying, cheating, and deceit. Sabotage is the deliberate destruction or interference with another person's production in order to gain competitive advantage. There are many, many forms of sabotage in academia. Subtle ways to derail someone's academic career include false accusations, vindictive personnel reviews, dishonest references, withholding information that someone needs to do their job, implicit biases, and sexual harassment. The perpetrator gains a competitive advantage while targets face criticism, skepticism, and blame. The target may eventually catch up for lost time in combatting false accusations. Unfortunately, the damage to reputation, self-esteem, and trust in colleagues does not recover to the pre-sabotage level. The loss of trust destroys the scientific community necessary to advance knowledge and human progress.

Because there are so many effective and discrete ways to sabotage a colleague, vandalizing experiments or data is rare. In order to interfere with data collection, the perpetrator must have unimpeded access to the experimental materials and knowledge of how to damage the experiment without getting caught. One such case occurred in 2011 when Mohsen Hosseinkhani was angry about losing his fellowship at Mount Sinai Medical Center in New York. He gained access to the lab and in the process of stealing $10,000 worth of stem-cell cultures, antibodies, and scientific equipment, Hosseinkhani stopped to mix up the experimental and control rats, a clear intention to mess with a colleague's experiment. Hosseinkhani was arrested and charged with burglary. Even though authorities had confiscated his passport for trial, Hosseinkhani fled to Iran and never faced charges. One of the better-documented cases of laboratory sabotage was experienced by Heather Ames as a graduate student at the University of Michigan in Ann Arbor.

Comprehensive Cancer Center, University of Michigan in Ann Arbor

Heather Ames was a graduate student in the Comprehensive Cancer Center at the University of Michigan in Ann Arbor. On December 12, 2009, Ames noticed a problem with her western blot assays. Four of her six samples were out of order. Initially, Ames thought she had made a mistake. When the problem occurred again five days later, Ames suspected that someone had switched the lids. She labelled her cultures on the bottom to avoid another incident. Next, Ames found an additional protein in her sample, an extra antibody. The events seemed to be a concerted effort to undermine her work. Her friends brushed her concerns aside, suggesting that she was paranoid. The cancer center researchers were a very professional team, supportive of one another. No one would sabotage a colleague's work. On Sunday, February 28, 2010, Ames noticed that her cell medium had an unusual consistency and odor. It smelled like alcohol. Ames took the medium to her supervisor who confirmed contamination. Ames's laboratory supervisor reported the issue to university administration.

Administration's initial response was that Ames was having difficulty in the laboratory and probably sabotaged her own work. Ames did not back down. After two more reports, the administrators called in public safety to investigate. University security focused their investigation on Ames. They interviewed Ames twice and had her take a lie detector test. On the morning of April 18, security officers installed hidden cameras in the lab. Ames worked in the lab as usual. The following day, her specimens were tainted again. When security reviewed the video, they observed postdoctoral student Vipul Bhrigu carrying a bottle of ethanol spray to the laboratory refrigerator and manipulating items within the refrigerator for over 30 seconds. Ames had never suspected Bhrigu. The postdoctoral student came to the United States from India, completed his PhD at the University of Toledo in Ohio, and earned a postdoctoral position in cancer research. Bhrigu was a postdoctoral student and Ames was only a graduate student. They were not in competition with one another. When security confronted Bhrigu with the evidence, he admitted tampering with Ames's samples in the video. He denied any involvement in the earlier incidents. He did admit to the recorded incident stating that he was trying to slow Ames down so that he could have a competitive advantage.

Bhrigu was charged with misdemeanor malicious destruction of personal property. The judge ordered a fine of $8,800 for damaged reagents and experimental materials, $600 in court fees, six months of probation, psychiatric evaluation, and 40 hours of community service. The prosecutor intended to sue for a further $72,000, compensating the university for losses due to salary and research time. Bhrigu fled to India before the second trial. Ames reported that there were times when the incidents caused her to want to leave science. Sabotage, no matter the form, wastes resources, erodes trust between scientists, and drives good people away. Fortunately, Ames's supervisor trusted her and was responsible enough to follow up on her reports. Many cases of sabotage go undetected or ignored by administrators.

STUDIES THAT "SHOULD NOT BE REPLICATED"

Some cases of scientific misconduct are revealed when other scientists are unable to replicate a published study. The Little Albert experiment, the Potti-Nevins studies (chapter 7), and Clever Hans could never be replicated. Then there are studies that should not be replicated, such as Kerr's killer bees or Aldini's electrical stimulation of a corpse. The Ig Nobel Prize awards originally started in 1991 as a way to celebrate "achievements that cannot or should not be reproduced." The awards are a tongue-in-cheek ceremony recognizing ridiculous, thought-provoking, or funny research and political achievements. Each year, the *Annals of Improbable Research*, Harvard-Radcliffe Society of Physics, and the Harvard-Radcliffe Science Fiction Association review 6,000–8,000 nominations to determine the recipients of 10 awards. The Ig Noble award ceremony is held in Sanders Theatre at Harvard University. Awards are given to the recipients by real Nobel Laureates. Notable awards include:

- James Cole, Zimbabwe, Tanzania, UK (Nutrition award, 2018) for determining that the caloric intake of the human-cannibalism diet is significantly lower than traditional meat diets.

- Jack Harvey, John Culvenor, Warren Payne, Steve Cowley, Michael Lawrence, David Stuart, and Robyn Williams, Australia (Physics award, 2003) for "An analysis of the forces required to drag sheep over various surfaces."

- K. P. Sreekumar and G. Nirmalan, Kerala Agricultural University, India (Mathematics award, 2002) for "Estimation of the total surface area in Indian elephants."

- Marie-Christine Cadiergues, Christel Joubert, and Michel Franc, Ecole Nationale Veterinaire de Toulouse, France (Biology award, 2008) for determining that fleas on dogs jump higher than fleas on cats.

- Catherine Bertenshaw [Douglas] and Peter Rowlinson, Newcastle University, UK (Veterinary Medicine award, 2009) for determining that cows with names produce more milk than cows without names.

- Anita Eerland and Rolf Zwaan, Utrecht University and Erasmus University, The Netherlands (Psychology award, 2012) for the study, "Leaning to the left makes the Eiffel Tower seem smaller."

- Francisco Alonso, Cristina Esteban, Andrea Serge, Maria-Luisa Ballestar, Jaime Sanmartín, Constanza Calatayud, and Beatriz Alamar, Spain, Columbia (Peace Prize, 2018) for their study, "Shouting and cursing while driving: Frequency, reasons, perceived risk and punishment."

- Christoph Helmchen, Carina Palzer, Thomas Münte, Silke Anders, and Andreas Sprenger, University of Luebeck, Germany (Medicine, 2016) for discovering that if you have an itch on one side of your body, you can relieve it by looking in a mirror and scratching the other side of your body.

- Evelyn Debbey, Maarten De Schryver, Gordon Logan, Kristina Suchotski, and Bruno Verschuere, Ghent University, Belgium (Psychology, 2016) "for asking a thousand liars how often they lie, and for deciding whether they believe those answers."

The Ig Nobel sponsors aim to recognize "achievements that make people LAUGH, and then THINK." Mostly, the Ig Nobel awards show that scientists have a sense of humor and not every experiment requires replication.

For many researchers, the major concerns during data collection are quality and calibration of the study instrument, identifying and responding appropriately to adverse events, and guarding against personal biases. Issues in data collection can jeopardize the health and welfare of study participants or invalidate study results. Who owns the samples or data, how the data will be used, and the long-term implications of data ownership continue to evolve in the legal, academic, and public arenas.

FURTHER READING

Bartels, Jared M., Marilyn M. Milovich, and Sabrina Moussier. 2016. "Coverage of the Stanford Prison Experiment in Introductory Psychology Courses." *Teaching of Psychology* 43 (2): 136–41.

"The BBC Prison Study." Accessed September 9, 2018. http://www.bbcprisonstudy.org/

Haslam, S. Alexander, Stephen D. Reicher, and Mark R. McDermott. 2015. "Studying Harm-Doing without Doing Harm: The Case of the BBC Prison Study, the Stanford Prison Experiment, and the Role-Conformity Model of Tyranny." In *Ethical Challenges in the Behavioral and Brain Sciences: Case Studies and Commentaries*, edited by Robert J. Sternberg and Susan T. Fiske, 134–39. New York: Cambridge University Press.

Heinzen, Thomas E., Scott O. Lilienfeld, and Susan A. Nolan. 2015. "Clever Hans." *Skeptic* 20 (1): 10–17.

Hubbard, Rebecca A., Karla Kerlikowske, Chris I. Flowers, Bonnie C. Yankaskas, Weiwei Zhu, and Diana L. Miglioretti. 2011. "Cumulative Probability of False-Positive Recall or Biopsy Recommendation after 10 Years of Screening Mammography: A Cohort Study." *Annals of Internal Medicine* 155 (8): 481–92.

Kaiser, Jocelyn. 2014. "Lab Incidents Lead to Safety Crackdown at CDC." *Science Now*, July 2. Accessed August 28, 2019. https://www.sciencemag.org/news/2014/07/lab-incidents-lead-safety-crackdown-cdc

Koppel, G., and N. Mirsky. 2002. *The Experiment*. British Broadcasting Corporation, May 14, 15, 20, 21.

Lehman, Constance D., Robert F. Arao, Brian L. Sprague, Janie M. Lee, Diana S. M. Buist, Karla Kerlikowske, Louise M. Henderson, et al. 2017. "National Performance Benchmarks for Modern Screening Digital Mammography: Update from the Breast Cancer Surveillance Consortium." *Radiology* 283 (1): 49–58.

Maher, Brendan. 2010. "Research Integrity: Sabotage!" *Nature* 467 (7315): 516–18.

Perry, Gina. 2018. "The Evil Inside Us All." *New Scientist* 240 (3199): 39–41.

Prakash, Snigdha, and Vikki Valentine. 2007. "Timeline: The Rise and Fall of Vioxx." *NPR*. Accessed January 24, 2019. https://www.npr.org/templates/story/story.php?storyId=5470430

Ratnesar, R. 2011. "The Menace Within." *Stanford Magazine*, July/August. Accessed January 3, 2019. https://stanfordmag.org/contents/the-menace -within

Skloot, Rebecca. 2010. *The Immortal Life of Henrietta Lacks*. New York: Crown Publishers.

Time-Life News Service. 1980. "The Big Sting." *Life* 3 (11): 79–84.

U.S. Department of Labor. n.d. "History of Federal Minimum Wage Rates under the Fair Labor Standards Act, 1938–2009." Accessed January 2, 2019. https://www.dol.gov/whd/minwage/chart.htm

Wilbur, Jason, and L. A. Carver. 2008. "Prostate Cancer Screening: The Continuing Controversy." *American Family Physician* 78 (12): 1377–84.

Zimbardo, Philip G. (1999–2019). "Stanford Prison Experiment." Accessed January 1, 2019. https://www.prisonexp.org/

SEVEN

Data Analysis and Drawing Conclusions

Once the researcher collects study data, the raw scores are converted into a form that is easier to understand. The first step in data analysis is *data cleaning*. *Data cleaning* is the process of identifying inaccurate, incomplete, or irrelevant data points and removing or correcting the data. *Data conversion* is the process of changing study data from one form to another, typically a format that allows the researcher and reader to easily draw conclusions. *Data analysis* is the process of inspecting, cleaning, converting, and examining the data in order to test the hypothesis, answer the research question, or draw conclusions. For example, a student achieves a raw score of 30 on an examination. Thirty sounds like an inferior grade until we learn that total possible points on the exam were 35 points. Converting 30 out of 35 to a percentage yields 85.7 percent. By converting the data, we conclude that the score is above average. How data are analyzed is determined by the research question or research hypothesis. With quantitative data, the researcher analyzes the data by descriptive or analytical statistics. Quantifiable results are calculated, analyzed, and presented in numerical, summarized form. For example, if the research hypothesis suggests that the experimental group will have higher scores on an outcome measure than the control group, the researcher analyzes the data to look at differences in the overall scores of both groups. If the research hypothesis suggests that two variables are related to one another, the researcher calculates the type and strength of relationship between two variables. Quantitative data are analyzed by statistical analysis. Qualitative data are analyzed by common themes or ideas. Qualitative data may be interviews, pictures, audio recording, x-ray images, or other nonnumerical data. The qualitative researcher reviews the data, codes the data, and draws conclusions. Both forms of data analysis look at patterns in the data. Much like data collection, data analysis is an area vulnerable to misconduct. Researchers work alone with very little oversight. If the data does not fit the expected results, the researcher may be tempted to throw out results that do not look right, or to fill in missing data points. Actions of concern are manipulating the data, removing outliers that do not support the hypothesis, reversing baseline and post-treatment results, filling in missing data, manipulating data, and over extrapolation of results.

HONEST ERROR

Everybody makes them—the dreaded math mistake—a decimal in the wrong place, reversing the plus or minus sign, or using the wrong unit. Math mistakes also happen to scientists. So much so that the definition of scientific misconduct specifically states, "research misconduct does not include honest error" (U.S. Department of Health and Human Services 2005). Common errors are problems with precise measurements, bad handwriting in laboratory notebooks, varying scientific units, tedious data entry, and errors in data transfer from one program to another. In 2015, PhD students at Tilburg University, Michèle B. Nuijten and Chris Hartgerink created Statcheck, a web-based program that checks for mathematical errors in APA formatted pdf files. The authors used Statcheck to analyze 30,717 articles published between 1985 and 2014 in eight major psychology journals (Nuijten et al. 2016). Fifty-four percent of the articles that tested for statistical significance contained a mathematical error and one in eight papers contained an error that could change the study conclusion. The researchers contacted all of the authors regarding the miscalculations and then published their findings on PubPeer, a website for people to discuss scientific research. The public disclosure through PubPeer was embarrassing for those who made mistakes. Some critics raised concerns about the accuracy of the program. Others were concerned with the possibility that public disclosure (or shaming) could harm public trust in science and scientists. Statcheck is now available for any researcher to upload and check calculations before publication. However, the program is limited to papers written in APA format. Statcheck is not the only service available for researchers to check calculations. There is a wide variety of online calculators available to help with complex mathematical calculations.

DATA FABRICATION

The three main types of scientific misconduct are data fabrication, data falsification, and plagiarism. Whereas falsification is the manipulation of results or omitting certain data points, data fabrication is the construction or addition of data that never occurred during an experiment. Basically, data fabrication is making up results. Fabrication may occur when the scientist needs to fill in data on a set of experiments or the scientist never successfully ran the experiments in the first place. Cases of data fabrication date back to the second century AD with Egyptian astronomer Claudius Ptolemy who claimed to perform measurements that he did not. Colleagues of Galileo Galilei also doubted that he ever performed some of his experiments. More recent cases of data fabrication include:

- **John Long**, researcher at Massachusetts General Hospital and Harvard Medical School. Long was awarded $759,000 to study cell cultures of patients with Hodgkin's disease. Suspicious colleagues inspected Long's cell cultures to find cell lines from the brown-footed Columbian owl monkey. Long resigned in 1980.

- **John Roland Darsee**, medical researcher at the Cardiac Research Laboratory, Harvard University worked on an NIH grant under world-renowned cardiologist Eugene Braunwald. Braunwald was so impressed by Darsee's prolific research and publishing that he offered Darsee a position at Brigham and Women's Hospital. Colleagues immediately raised concerns about Darsee's experiments. Believing that the work in question was an isolated incident, Braunwald rescinded the job offer but did not notify the NIH. When Darsee's data did not match results from other study sites, a university committee was assembled to investigate. Investigators found substantial evidence of data fabrication dating back to Darsee's time as an undergraduate at the University of Notre Dame. The NIH criticized Braunwald for not reporting, barred Darsee from attaining NIH funding for 10 years, and ordered Brigham and Women's Hospital to repay $122,371 in research funding. Darsee's case was the first time an institution was required to pay back research funds resulting from misconduct. In 1984, the state of New York pulled Darsee's medical license. He currently works under an alias as a medical writer designing training programs for pharmaceutical sales representatives and physicians.

- **Steven Breuning**, psychologist and clinical director of the Polk Center in Pennsylvania published research showing that Ritalin was more effective than tranquilizers in treating children with intellectual disabilities. In 1983, Breuning sent Robert Sprague of the University of Illinois an abstract describing a two-year study with biannual follow-ups of 45 of 57 participants who had previously taken part in a Breuning study at Coldwater Center. Sprague knew that the numbers and the dates did not line up with Breuning's employment at Coldwater Center. Sprague reported his concerns to the study funder, the NIMH and quickly found himself the focus of investigation. Despite 17 years of continuous funding, the NIMH stopped Sprague's funding. In 1988, Breuning was found guilty of misappropriating federal funds and sentenced to 60 days on work release, 250 hours of community service, 5 years' probation, and required to repay part of his salary from the period of misconduct.

- **Dipak Das**, director of the Cardiovascular Research Center at the University of Connecticut Health Center is best known for his research on the effects of red wine on heart disease. In 2005, a university committee questioned how Das obtained certain measurements when no one in the laboratory had the technical expertise to perform such analyses. By the time the investigation was complete, the committee found 145 cases of data fabrication!

- **Woo Suk Hwang** was professor of veterinary medicine at Seoul National University when he reported successfully cloning human stem cells from patients with spinal cord injuries and other diseases. Hwang became a national hero. Embryonic stem cells have the ability to become any type of cell in the body. Stem cell treatment could potentially replace malfunctioning or injured cells with genetically matched clone cells. In 2005, Hwang announced plans for a clinical trial, replacing the nerve cells of a 10-year-old boy with spinal cord injury. Young-Joon Ryu was a former employee and lead researcher on Hwang's initial trials. He left Hwang's lab in 2004 to work at the Korea Cancer Center Hospital. Ryu knew Hwang's studies were not as they appeared to be and he feared for the boy's health. Ryu contacted Munhwa Broadcasting Corporation and recommended an investigation. Hwang's supporters attacked and threatened Ryu. His wife and eight-month-old daughter had to go into hiding for six months. In 2006, Hwang admitted using cells from IVF embryos. He was found guilty of embezzling 830 million won (~$700,000) and buying human eggs in violation of South Korean law.

- **Diederick Stapel**, professor of social psychology at Tilburg University, the University of Groningen, and the University of Amsterdam worked with students to plan research studies and then created fictitious research assistants who purportedly collected data from middle school students. Investigation found that Stapel published at least 30 peer-reviewed papers based on fabricated or manipulated data. In 2011, Stapel voluntarily returned his doctorate to the University of Amsterdam. The website Retraction Watch lists 54 retractions associated with Stapel's misconduct.

- **Anil Potti**, associate professor of medicine at Duke University studied genomic medicine in cancer treatment. In 2006, Potti and his supervisor, Joseph Nevins, published a study claiming that the gene activity of cancer cells could be used to determine the most effective chemotherapy for each individual patient. Researchers at M. D. Anderson Cancer Center of the University of Texas attempted to replicate the study results without success.

After back and forth discussion between the two groups, the Potti-Nevins team sent the M. D. Anderson group their data. The data contained serious errors. In some cases, cell lines were reversed meaning the patients received the least effective therapy rather than the most effective therapy. The two groups continued to share data and the M. D. Anderson researchers kept finding numerous mistakes. When they attempted to submit their concerns to the journals publishing the Potti-Nevins studies, their correspondence was rejected without explanation. In 2015, a third-year medical student working with Potti and Nevins, Bradford Perez, became concerned with his supervisors' study methods and contacted Duke University officials. The officials referred Perez to Nevins. Perez requested that his name be withdrawn as contributor on four papers, a very bold move for a medical student who could benefit greatly with publications on his resume. After other researchers were unable to replicate the Potti-Nevins results, the National Cancer Institute (NCI) started an investigation. The investigators found multiple false achievements on Potti's resume, such as claiming to be a Rhodes scholar. In 2015, a full investigation by the Office of Research Integrity found Potti had fabricated, reversed, and falsified data. Nevins was criticized for advocating for Potti to university officials. Ten publications by Potti-Nevins were retracted based on the falsified data. In a further bizarre twist of events, Retraction Watch, a blog that reports retracted scientific papers was the target of a Digital Millennium Copyright Act (DMCA) takedown notice. Retraction Watch was accused of plagiarizing their report of Potti by a website in India. The website had actually plagiarized from Retraction Watch and then filed a complaint against Retraction Watch. Potti denied being behind the false claim. WordPress.org was hit with a similar accusation on their content related to Potti. The complaint demanded that they take down their report on Potti.

- **Dong-Pyou Han**, vaccine researcher and assistant professor of biomedical sciences at Iowa State University, added human blood to rabbit blood to make it look like his HIV vaccine exhibited stronger activity than it actually did. In 2014, Han was arrested on four counts of felony. He was ordered to repay $7.2 million to the NIH and sentenced to 57 months in prison with three years of supervised release.

- **Scott S. Reuben** was professor of anesthesiology and pain management at Tufts University in Boston and chief of acute pain at Baystate Medical Center. Over 13 years, Reuben published 21 articles reporting clinical efficacy of pain management drugs. His reports always showed favorable results for the pharmaceutical company funding the trial. Experts estimate that Reuben's research produced billions of dollars for pharmaceutical companies. Authorities started asking questions when Reuben planned to present study results for research that had never been reviewed by Baystate's research review board. On investigation, Reuben admitted fabricating patients and study results. In 2010, Reuben was convicted of healthcare fraud, sentenced to six months in federal prison with three years' supervised release, and ordered to pay $360,000 restitution plus a $5,000 fine.

With so many cases of data fabrication, the question of why arises. Why would a person risk professional career, reputation, years of education, freedom, and financial stability? Wouldn't it be easier just to do the research? A review of the cases suggests scientists are tempted to fabricate data when faced with severe pressure to produce groundbreaking research or when they believe they already know the answer and taking the time to collect data seems unnecessary. The temptation is compounded by arrogance, laziness, greed, corrupted power, or incompetence. The lack of oversight seems to play a major role in data fabrication. The number of whistle-blowers who were subjected to investigation, rebuke, or punishment for expressing concerns is concerning since failure to report would have implicated them in each scandal.

Painting the Mice

The case of data fabrication by William Summerlin deserves special mention because his technique was stunningly simple and resulted in the term *painting the mice*, a metaphor for data fabrication. Dr. William Talley Summerlin was a researcher at Sloan Kettering Cancer Center in New York City. While a student at Stanford University School of Medicine, Summerlin reportedly developed a special medical technique to promote successful tissue and organ transplantation. Transplantation is a form of treatment for patients suffering from severe burns or organ failure. With tissue transplants, there is a high chance that the recipient's body will identify the donor tissue as a foreign body and attack and kill the transplanted cells, a process known as rejection. Drugs are given to suppress the immune response, thereby forcing the recipient's body to accept the transplanted tissue. Immune suppression increases the recipient's susceptibility to deadly infections. Summerlin's discovery was a breakthrough in the science of organ transplant because it reduced the need for immunosuppressive therapy.

Given his amazing success and potential for groundbreaking research, the rising star moved to Memorial Sloan Kettering Cancer Center in New York City where he became the chief of transplant immunology. In July 1973, Summerlin reported that he had successfully transplanted skin grafts from black mice onto white mice using a special laboratory technique. His technique consisted of culturing the donated tissue before transplant, allowing cells that would trigger the immune reaction to "migrate" out of the graft. On March 27, 1974, James Martin was working as a laboratory assistant in Summerlin's lab. He was handling the recipient mouse when he noticed black marks on his hand. The black coloring came from the recipient mouse. Martin wiped the "graft" with alcohol to reveal the mouse's original white fur. The laboratory assistants reported their discovery to Sloan Kettering administration. To his credit, Summerlin admitted using a black felt tip marker to create the image of transplanted tissue. In his defense, Summerlin claimed that he was under immense job strain. He was unable to meet the pressures of the position and research deadlines. He created the impression of a successful transplant to placate demands. Sloan Kettering administrators found evidence of data fabrication in Summerlin's earlier studies at Stanford and recommended dismissal. Summerlin was placed on one year of paid leave while he obtained mental health treatment (Basu 2006).

DATA CLEANING

To clean the data, the scientist looks at the data, either by individual participants or as summary data, and considers whether the recorded data are accurate or make sense. For example, in a study of physical activity, the researcher might collect data on daily step count from 99 participants over the period of one month. Participant 45 reported daily step counts normally ranging from 4,000 to 15,000 steps per day. On Day 6, this participant recorded 102,859 steps. Clearly, 102,000 steps is either a huge outlier or an error in recording. If the researcher is able to go back and verify 102,000 steps with the participant or through electronic recording, the data point may be calculated along with the other results. If the number cannot be verified, the researcher would consider removing the questionable data point from the final analysis. Trying to guess at what the number should have been creates too many questions and concerns with data manipulation. Data cleaning is part of good research practice. Problems occur when the researcher throws out too many outliers or purposely selects data to remove in order to strengthen support for the hypothesis. One example of this is parapsychologist Joseph Banks Rhine. While studying telepathy and clairvoyance, Rhine tossed out low scores claiming study participants were intentionally giving the wrong answers. In clinical research, data manipulation can have devastating effects, such as the ghostwriter who fudged the data from Study 329 (chapter 3) leading to the death of several young adults taking Paxil for depression. In the 1990s, a Wyeth safety officer overwrote computer files to erase evidence that the diet drug Fen-Phen caused heart and lung problems. Approximately 5.8 million people, mostly young healthy women, took Fen-Phen. Many suffered long-lasting effects. More than 50,000 victims filed lawsuits against Wyeth. In 2006, Wyeth settled for over $22 billion.

A second issue with data cleaning is overzealous cleaning. Human beings vary. Study samples vary. A research participant's step counts will not be exactly the same on each day or the same as other participants in the study. Despite this basic principle of human nature, there have been cases in history where scientists reported data that were simply too good to be true. Reviewers believe that geneticist Gregor Mendel threw out beans that did not favor his hypothesis on dominant and recessive genes. Physicist Robert Millikan may have doctored his results in order to minimize questions and disagreements by colleagues. Data that are too good to be true are often revealed during secondary analysis, as was the case of Anil Potti at Duke University. Data manipulation is a slippery slope. The more one engages in misconduct, the easier it becomes, until someone eventually detects the problem.

The Longitudinal Study of Aging

Eric T. Poehlman was a highly respected tenured professor at the University of Vermont (UVM) College of Medicine. He published over 200 articles on his research specialty, obesity, exercise, and aging. He enjoyed one of the highest salaries of the university. Students loved the smart, athletic, and personable professor who was known to spend recreational time with his graduate assistants. When Walter DeNino was invited to work in Poehlman's laboratory, he was thrilled. DeNino planned to attend medical school. A year working as a laboratory assistant would provide valuable research experience and the opportunity to publish with a world-renowned scientist. The experience would make his medical school application stand out. DeNino joined an existing project entitled The Longitudinal Study of Aging. He was responsible for statistical analysis of cholesterol, triglycerides, high density lipoproteins (HDL), and low density lipoproteins (LDL) blood levels of the study volunteers.

Poehlman instructed DeNino to get the current data spreadsheet from a former member of the team who had moved to Canada. The contact did not respond immediately. In the meantime, DeNino learned that another member of the project team, someone right down the hall, also had a copy of the spreadsheet. DeNino obtained the spreadsheet and started analyzing the data. He noticed that the data did not match the anticipated changes in triglycerides, HDL, and LDL levels. Results were not statistically significant and instead of the expected decrease in total cholesterol, there was an increase. DeNino showed his analysis results to Poehlman. A week later, Poehlman returned the spreadsheet to DeNino with instructions to re-analyze the data. On the second analysis, DeNino found that the study results supported Poehlman's hypothesis. DeNino was confused and compared the three spreadsheets, the original, the one that had finally arrived from Canada, and the one provided by Poehlman. He found that lab values on Poehlman's spreadsheet were edited. When he asked Poehlman about the edits, Poehlman explained that he had corrected data entry errors. This explanation did not make sense. Errors in data entry would be random with some values supporting the hypothesis and other values not supporting the hypothesis. Poehlman's edits all supported the hypothesis.

DeNino confided in a former staff member of Poehlman's laboratory, Dr. Andre Tchernof. Tchernof confirmed DeNino's concerns noting that there had been questions in the past about Poehlman's study data. He warned DeNino to be careful. Poehlman had a history of getting nasty with laboratory assistants who questioned his results. Tchernof pointed out that DeNino was in a lose-lose situation. If he kept quiet, he could be involved in data fabrication, a serious breach of research integrity. If he reported his concerns, he could be guilty of making a false accusation against a well-respected scientist and popular professor. On the other hand, the finding of data fabrication could end the professor's career as well as his own. As DeNino struggled with his conscience, he consulted a second colleague. The colleague also cautioned against reporting and recommended that if DeNino did decide to report, he should collect evidence to support his report. DeNino went back to the original patient charts and checked the lab results against Poehlman's spreadsheet. He found that among patients where blood levels improved, Poehlman switched the values to make it look like the values had gotten worse. Where data were missing, Poehlman made up results. If the changes in lab values were not large enough to show statistical difference, Poehlman adjusted the numbers to support statistical significance. There was a clear pattern of purposeful changes.

DeNino approached Dr. Burton E. Sobel, chair of the department of medicine. Sobel confronted Poehlman who initially dismissed the accusation. Since Poehlman had received federal funding for his research, the University of Vermont feared they would be implicated in fraud. Per protocol, the University of Vermont started a formal investigation. Poehlman offered multiple conflicting explanations for the altered data. He claimed that (1) the original values were errors in data entry, (2) the file became corrupted when his hard drive crashed, (3) his values were imputed or predicted values, (4) other members of the team had inadvertently created errors in the data set, (5) the revised data were simulated to test various scenarios, (6) the irregularities were computer error, and (7) a laboratory worker had falsified the data and sent the falsified data from Poehlman's e-mail account. During the investigation, Poehlman attempted to destroy electronic evidence. He moved to the University of Montreal where he was later asked to leave. As his explanations shifted, Poehlman attacked DeNino. With limited funds from his laboratory assistant position, DeNino was forced to hire a lawyer for his own legal defense (Interlandi 2006).

Joint investigations by the University of Vermont and U.S. Department of Health and Human Services Office of Research Integrity revealed that the research misconduct in The Longitudinal Study on Aging was just the tip of the iceberg. From about 1992 to 2000, Poehlman fabricated results in three research studies and published 10 articles with fabricated data. Of the 35 participants reported in Poehlman's The Longitudinal Menopause Study (1994–2000), Poehlman made up results for 32 participants. In The Prospective Hormone Replacement Therapy Study (1999–2000), Poehlman did not even have access to the data and simply fabricated results. As evidence mounted and excuses exhausted, Poehlman pled guilty to making material false statements in federal grant applications. In the final university report, it was determined that Poehlman used fake data to apply for 17 federal government grants worth approximately $11.6 million. He was awarded $2.9 million in grants. Under legal settlement, Poehlman agreed to reimburse the federal government $180,000, cover DeNino's legal fees of $16,000, and to retract all articles with fabricated data. He is barred for life from seeking funding from any federal agency, including Medicare, Medicaid, or other federal health care programs. Under federal sentencing guidelines, Poehlman could have served up to five years in prison for defrauding the federal government. He served one year and one day in prison with two years of probation. Poehlman was the first American scientist to serve prison time for research fraud.

Joachim Boldt

Joachim Boldt was a well-known and well-respected anesthesiologist and researcher at Klinikum Ludwigshafen, a large teaching hospital in Germany. Most of Boldt's research investigated the intravenous use of hetastarch (hydroxyethylene starch, HES) to expand blood volume and support blood pressure during and after surgery. Hetastarch products are controversial. They may cause kidney failure. Boldt co-authored numerous studies with other prominent anesthesiologists. The studies showed that a colloidal form of hetastarch was safe. Based on the research, medical societies issued guidelines endorsing the use of colloidal hetastarch. In December 2009, *Anesthesia and Analgesia* published a study by Boldt comparing hetastarch and albumin. After the publication, journal editor Stephen Shafer received an e-mail questioning the study data. The letter writer noted surprise over the small study sample, very small standard deviation, and high statistical significance. With normal human variation, it is difficult to get high levels of significance from small study samples. Shafer was not concerned. The article had gone through two peer reviews. A second letter arrived the next day also raising concerns. Shafer contacted Boldt for clarification and read the article a third time. This time he noticed a perfect acid-base balance report. Mechanical ventilation, fluid loss during surgery, intravenous fluid replacement, kidney function and cellular respiration all influence acid-base balance. To attain a perfect acid-base balance post-surgery is nearly impossible. Boldt did not respond to Shafer's requests for clarification.

Eventually, Shafer contacted the state medical association, Landesärztekammer Rheinland-Pfalz (LAK-RLP). LAK-RLP investigated and found no evidence that the study patients existed. There was no record of study review by the Rheinland-Pfalz review board and Klinikum Ludwigshafen had no record of administering albumin to patients after 1999. *Anesthesia and Analgesia* retracted the article. Boldt admitted forging the signatures of co-authors. He was fired by the hospital and his co-authors were fired for refusing to cooperate with the investigation. By 2011, the LAK-RLP and hospital investigators reviewed 74 journal articles and found no ethical approval for 68 of Boldt's studies. In 2013, external reviewers analyzed 38 clinical studies of HES (Zarychanski et al. 2013). Including Boldt's studies in the analysis, patients who received HES were at 1.07 times higher risk for death. Excluding Boldt's studies, patients who received HES were at a 1.09 times higher risk for death, 1.27 times higher risk of renal failure, and 1.32 times higher risk for renal replacement fluid. The researchers concluded that patients receiving HES were at significantly greater risk for kidney injury and death. Ninety-six of Boldt's articles were withdrawn from the anesthesia literature, the most retractions of any individual.

Boldt's studies significantly influenced anesthesia practices and policies and put patients' lives at risk. German authorities were determining whether to press criminal charges when Boldt left Germany. He is believed to be working in the Czech Republic as an anesthetist. Shafer believes Boldt's main motive for the deceit was vanity and self-promotion. Boldt was considered a world expert in anesthesiology. Companies flew him first class around the world and treated him to lavish meals and expenses so that he would attend or speak at their conferences. Based on the experience with Boldt, *Anesthesia and Analgesia* implemented a series of procedures to ensure better oversight and review of published studies.

BIG DATA, DATA DREDGING, AND SALAMI SLICING

Big data refers to large data sets. Large data sets are electronic databases that require special software tools to capture, manage, process, and analyze data. Examples in health care include disease registries, electronic medical records, health insurance records, prescription plans, retail transactions, or motor vehicle crash records. Large data sets are particularly useful because researchers can search a vast amount of data very quickly and relatively inexpensively. The data are already collected, saving hours and years of data collection. Any data collected by tax dollars falls under the purview of public access, which means de-identified data may be accessed free of charge. Another advantage of big data is that missing data can be filled in with statistically appropriate, projected numbers.

The main function of big data in research is to test relationships. This usage presents problems. Statistical significance is dependent on the results, sample size, and confidence interval, an estimate of the population parameter. With large samples, very small differences may appear statistically significant because of the large sample size. Chapter 4 describes how Tyler Vigen used big data to analyze numerous farcical correlations. Vigen found a significant positive correlation between the number of letters in the winning word of Scripps National Spelling Bee and the number of people killed by venomous spiders ($r = 0.8057$). Based on Vigen's analysis, one might conclude that the venomous spiders are angry about the number of letters in the winning words of the Scripps National Spelling Bee and are attacking people or the Scripps National Spelling Bee leads to an increased population of venomous spiders. Common sense tells us that the two variables are not related. The result is a false positive. However, relationships are not always clear especially if the person doing the analysis has an agenda. *Data mining* can mislead people into thinking there is a significant relationship between two variables when there is not. More contemptuous terms for data mining are data dredging, data fishing, or p-hacking. P-hacking is a reference to p value or probability, the statistical notation enumerating significance of the results. In social sciences, a p value of less than .05 is statistically significant. A p value of less than .05 means that the results will only occur by chance less than 5 times out of 100. With large data sets, it is easier to get statistically significant p values. There is the potential to abuse big data by repeatedly checking statistical significance with selected variables or finding statistically significant results and then developing a post-hoc hypothesis. Data fishing damages scientific credibility, misleads other researchers and scientific progress, and wastes valuable research funding. The best way to avoid data dredging is to have a clear and sensible plan for data analysis outlined in the research protocol and to stick with the plan.

Salami slicing is when the researcher breaks up a large data set into smaller sets and tests the same or a very similar hypothesis in order to create multiple articles. The practice, also known as Least Publishable Unit (LPU), loot, and publons, is common among early-career researchers who need several publications by the time of tenure and promotion review or are trying to inflate the number of publications for grant applications. However, there are certainly many mid- to late career researchers who also engage in salami slicing. The practice values number of publications over quality of publications. For example, one large data set of 1,000 study participants could be reported in a top-tier journal or sliced into smaller sets of approximately 200 study participants to yield five publications in lower tier journals. Alternatively, a researcher might separate questions on a lengthy survey into smaller sets and publish different aspects of the survey. The advantage of salami slicing is that it allows early career researchers to publish work in stages rather than waiting years for final results. Working with smaller data sets is less overwhelming than one large data set. LPU articles are also a symbol of progress, a sign that the researcher is overcoming self-doubt and self-criticism to successfully build a research agenda. Disadvantages of salami slicing are that in reducing the size of the study sample, variation increases and statistically significant results are weaker. If the researcher writes articles based on the same research hypothesis, it is difficult not to use similar wording or terms. Salami slicing can easily become self-plagiarism. The practice of LPU creates problems for other scientists. In reviewing the literature, LPU's will make it look like there are more studies on a particular phenomenon than there actually are. An excessive number of papers from one study or one source is misleading to reviewers and practitioners.

PREMATURE OR OVEREXTRAPOLATION OF RESULTS

Extrapolation is a statistical tool for finding a particular value outside of a set of data. In clinical trials, scientists often extrapolate data between adults and children. If a particular disease demonstrates the same clinical progression in children as in adults and response to intervention is similar, researchers might extrapolate the study results using treatments that are effective among adults to treat children. Extrapolation reduces the number of clinical trials among children, saving time and resources. *Premature extrapolation* refers to estimating values before the final results are known or confirmed. Premature extrapolation would be assuming that a treatment may be used in children before final testing in adults. *Overextrapolation* refers to estimating values beyond known data. Overextrapolation would be assuming the treatment works for people with similar health issues. Premature extrapolation and overextrapolation stretch the boundaries of reason. The 1977 study of saccharin in laboratory rats is a good example of overextrapolation of results and the dangers of overextrapolation.

Artificial Sweeteners and Cancer in Laboratory Rats

Saccharin was discovered unintentionally in 1879. The artificial sweetener quickly grew in popularity and use. It could make medicines more palatable, sweeten food for diabetics or others on low sugar diets, help with food preservation, and disguise inferior products. However, there was never any formal safety testing. As saccharin and other food substitutes became more common, people started to question safety. In 1977, a group of researchers published a study indicating that saccharin caused bladder cancer in laboratory rats. The researchers extrapolated their results to humans warning that saccharin could cause bladder cancer. News agencies immediately reported the study. The National Cancer Institute advised the public not to ingest saccharin. The federal government listed saccharin as a carcinogen. A warning label was applied to all products containing saccharin. As other researchers attempted to replicate the study, they found that rats have a unique mechanism of metabolizing saccharin. Humans do not have the same biological mechanism. Saccharin does not cause bladder cancer in humans. Despite subsequent experiments, it took almost 20 years for the federal government to remove saccharin from the list of carcinogens.

STATISTICAL SIGNIFICANCE VERSUS PRACTICAL SIGNIFICANCE

Researchers often become so focused on statistical significance that they forget about practical significance of the results. In quantitative research, study results that meet the level of statistical significance are deemed important. Results that do not reach statistical significance are deemed unimportant. In the real world, statistical significance is simply a number. Practical significance or clinical significance is what is most important. Imagine there is a disease affecting newborns where the newborns die within an hour of birth. A new treatment extends the life of newborns with this horrific disease to 24 hours. Increasing life span from one hour to 24 hours is statistically significant. However, the result is still the same. Infants still die from the disease. The treatment has limited practical significance. Practical significance relates to real life. Practical significance tells us whether the results truly make a difference.

Within the scope of scientific misconduct, data analysis seems to be the stage where too many scientists falter and fail. Working in isolation allows individuals to engage in data fabrication or data falsification. The reasons for corruption may be narcissism, where the perpetrator is sure that he or she already knows the results and does not need to spend time on experimentation, lack of ability to make the experiment work, or laziness. Eventually, those who fabricate data will get caught when other scientists attempt to replicate the original study and are unable to. The problem is that in the meantime, research funding is exploited, other scientists waste valuable time, study participants undergo unnecessary procedures, and the general public is misled or loses faith in science. Best practices in laboratory record-keeping and adequate oversight by laboratory supervisors and administrators can prevent some scientific misconduct during the data collection stage of a study.

FURTHER READING

Agin, Dan. 2006. *Junk science: How Politicians, Corporations, and Other Hucksters Betray Us*. New York: Thomas Dunne Books.

Arnold, D. L., C. A. Moodie, B. Stavric, D. R. Stoltz, H. C. Grice, and I. C. Munro. 1977. "Canadian Saccharin Study." *Science* (4301): 320–320.

Basu, Paroma. 2006. "Where Are They Now?" *Nature Medicine* 12 (5): 492–93.

Culliton, Barbara J. 1977. "Saccharin: A Chemical in Search of an Identity." *Science* 196 (4295): 1179–183.

Dahlberg, John E., and Christian C. Mahler. 2006. "The Poehlman Case: Running Away from the Truth." *Science & Engineering Ethics* 12 (1): 157–73.

Hicks, R. M., J. S. Wakefield, and J. Chowaniec. 1973. "Co-carcinogenic Action of Saccharin in the Chemical Induction of Bladder Cancer." *Nature* 243 (5406): 347–49.

Interlandi, Jeneen. 2006. "An Unwelcome Discovery." *New York Times Magazine*, October 22, 98–114.

Mundy, Alicia. 2001. *Dispensing with the Truth: The Victims, the Drug Companies, and the Dramatic Story behind the Battle over Fen-Phen*. London: St. Martin's Press.

Nuijten, Michèle B., Chris H. J. Hartgerink, Marcel A. L. M. van Assen, Sacha Epskamp, and Jelte M. Wicherts. 2016. "The Prevalence of Statistical Reporting Errors in Psychology (1985–2013)." *Behavior Research Methods* 48 (4): 1205–26.

Smart, Pippa. 2017. "Redundant Publication and Salami Slicing: The Significance of Splitting Data." *Developmental Medicine & Child Neurology* 59 (8): 775–775.

Statcheck. Accessed November 21, 2019. http://statcheck.io/index.php

Szucs, Denes. 2016. "A Tutorial on Hunting Statistical Significance by Chasing N." *Frontiers in Psychology* 7. doi:10.3389/fpsyg.2016.01444

Tilden, Samuel J. 2010. "Incarceration, Restitution, and Lifetime Debarment: Legal Consequences of Scientific Misconduct in the Eric Poehlman Case." *Science & Engineering Ethics* 16 (4): 737–41.

U.S. Department of Health and Human Services. 2005. "Federal Register: 42 CFR Part 93." Accessed June 11, 2018. https://ori.hhs.gov/sites/default/files/42_cfr_parts_50_and_93_2005.pdf

U.S. Department of Health and Human Services. Office of Research Integrity. n.d. "Case summary—Eric T. Poehlman." Accessed June 11, 2018. https://ori.hhs.gov/case-summary-eric-t-poehlman

Wise, Jacqui. 2013. "Boldt: The Great Pretender." *British Medical Journal* 346 (7900): 16–18.

Zarychanski, Ryan, Ahmed M. Abou-Setta, Alexis F. Turgeon, Brett L. Houston, Lauralyn McIntyre, John C. Marshall, and Dean A. Fergusson. 2013. "Association of Hydroxyethyl Starch Administration with Mortality and Acute Kidney Injury in Critically Ill Patients Requiring Volume Resuscitation." *JAMA: Journal of the American Medical Association* 309 (7): 678–88.

EIGHT

Communicating Study Findings

Once a study is completed, the researchers have a professional responsibility to share results with interested study participants, funders, peers, policy makers, patients, communities, and news journalists. Peer scientists are eager to learn of other colleagues' research and results. Shared knowledge allows the scientific field to advance. If scientists kept study findings to themselves, human progress would slow or halt. The standard progression of dissemination of information is (1) presentation at professional conferences to others working in the discipline, (2) professional journals, (3) professional organizations, (4) media outlets, and (5) the public. This progression starts with those who are highly invested in the topic, scientific peers, and moves to the wider audience of interested groups. Sharing knowledge allows scientists to learn and plan ways to further investigate the phenomenon of interest.

Initially, colleagues in the field present study findings at conferences and in peer-to-peer discussions. The audience provides feedback on whether study results make sense and whether the conclusions seem accurate and logical. This peer review also allows other scientists to validate results. Peer review and replication provide a system of checks and balances. Independent testing by other scientists is a way to confirm accuracy of the original study and possible modification of study procedures for future investigation. In theory, if the study results are flawed, peers should be able to detect errors either by looking at the results or in trying to replicate the study. The typical venues for peer review are professional conferences and scientific journal publications. Each professional association holds regular conferences to share the latest research, practices, tools, and technologies. For example, the American Public Health Association holds an annual conference that attracts almost 13,000 researchers, practitioners, policy makers, and other people each year. Researchers submit short overviews of their research to the conference organizers who then read and rank presentations based on relevance to the conference and interest to the audience. Presentations vary from 10 minutes to an hour followed by questions and comments from the audience. This review process and subsequent discussion help scientists to understand where other scientists might have questions or concerns regarding the study. Peer critique strengthens current and future projects for both the scientist and reviewers.

Professional organizations partner with publishers to print and distribute peer-reviewed journals. For example, the American Public Health Association manages the *American Journal of Public Health* (*AJPH*). The American Medical Association manages the *Journal of the American Medical Association* (*JAMA*) as well as 13 other professional journals for specialty practitioners. Publishing in a top-tier professional, peer-reviewed journal is the goal of many researchers. Successful publication demonstrates that the scientist made an important contribution to the field. Publication brings recognition and expands opportunities for grants and further research. However, it is not easy to publish in prestigious professional journals. Acceptance rates are low. *JAMA* editors receive more than 4,400 research submissions each year and only 4 percent are published. To publish a research study in a scholarly journal, the researcher must identify the appropriate journal for publication, write a manuscript that meets the venue's publication criteria, and submit the manuscript for review. Outside reviewers read, comment on, and score the manuscript giving a final recommendation of (a) publish as is, (b) edit for publication, or (c) reject. The goal of peer review is to help editors determine whether submissions are worthy of publication. The system is not fail-safe. For example, to test peer reviewer abilities, editors of the *British Medical Journal* intentionally inserted eight errors in a manuscript and sent it to 420 potential reviewers (Godlee, Gale, and Martyn 1998). Two hundred and twenty-one reviewers responded. The median number of mistakes caught was two, none of the reviewers identified more than five, and 16 percent did not identify any mistakes. Peer review is designed to determine the merits of publication, not to detect fraudulent activity or research misconduct. The challenges of peer review deter some researchers. Predatory journals have become a way to bypass peer review and therefore the system of checks and balances that aims to limit bad science (see chapter 3).

Dissemination in the popular media typically comes after professional dissemination and peer review. Examples of popular media are the internet, newspapers, magazines, books, television, or videos. If the research findings are of interest to the public, a researcher may contact the media to disseminate results. Working with the press requires different skills than presenting at a professional conference or publishing. With the press, the scientist often has only a few seconds to convey a meaningful message. Translating complex scientific information into brief, understandable sound bites is challenging. Existing beliefs or biases against science and scientists may influence the way the audience receives the message. Audiences may be put off by scientists who appear boring, challenge current beliefs, or seem out of touch with reality. When messages are not consistent with what the public wants to hear, the scientist can become the target of vicious backlash. Overly eager scientists, poor journalism practices and public response can allow poorly researched or sensational stories to make the news without any consideration for the truth.

THE PEER REVIEW PROCESS

Peer reviewers are supposed to be experts in their field who are able to read a manuscript, identify strengths and weaknesses, suggest edits, and advise editors on whether to publish. The task is unpaid. Reviewers volunteer their time and effort as service to the professional community. To support unbiased reviews, editors remove author names. Anonymous reviews allow the reviewer to focus on content rather than title, gender, or reputation of the researcher. With legitimate professional journals, two or three peer reviewers review each manuscript. Peer review can be a difficult process for the reviewer and the reviewee. *Discover* magazine offers revealing insight into the peer review process through their 2010 list of favorite quotes from peer reviewers:

> "This paper is desperate. Please reject it completely and then block the author's e-mail ID so they can't use the online system in the future."
>
> "The biggest problem with this manuscript, which has nearly sucked the will to live out of me, is the terrible writing style."
>
> "I agreed to review this MS [manuscript] while answering e-mails in the golden glow of a balmy evening on the terrace of our holiday hotel on Lake Como. Back in the harsh light of reality in Belfast I realize that it's just on the limit of my comfort zone and that it would probably have been better not to have volunteered." (Welsh 2010)

The peer review process can take up to several months. Because the process is resource intensive, authors must agree not to submit the manuscript to other journals. Editors do not want to waste reviewer time and expertise giving feedback on a paper only for the article to be published somewhere else. Authors may only submit to other journals if their paper is rejected. The peer process can be even more painful for the researcher who has spent years on a study only to be told that results are not worthy of publication. There are many reasons for rejection, for example, results are not statistically significant, study methods were not rigorous, writing style is unclear, or the topic is not a good fit with the journal. It can take years to get a research study published in a professional journal.

Given the hurdles of peer review, it is not surprising that many would-be authors will go to great lengths to bypass peer review. In China, the government funds most of the research. In order to gain funding, researchers must publish in high impact journals. The pressure to publish has resulted in many high-profile cases of scientific misconduct. In 2007, the Ministry of Science and Technology (MST) identified 486 cancer researchers engaging in a fraudulent peer-review scheme. The investigation resulted in retraction of 107 papers from *Tumor Biology*, the most papers retracted by one journal. In 2015, editors of the *British Journal of Clinical Pharmacology* were forced to examine their peer review process. The editors received a manuscript reporting a meta-analysis comparing mortality of recombinant brain natriuretic peptide (Rhbnp) and the drug dobutamine. The authors suggested two peer reviewers, both well-known experts at Ivy League institutions in the United States. The normal editorial practice was to use one suggested reviewer and a second reviewer from the peer reviewer pool. In this case, the editors decided to use both of the suggested reviewers. Requests for reviews were sent and within a day, both reviewers agreed. The reviews were completed and returned within four days, an incredible turnaround time for busy working professionals. Peer review statements were positive suggesting only minor edits. After publication, a journal club selected the article for discussion. Club members found multiple errors and wrote a detailed letter to the editor. Disturbed by the number of mistakes raised by the group, the editors went back to the peer reviews. In examining the peer review comments, the editors realized that the peer reviews contained poor grammar and the reviewers' e-mail addresses were not associated with their work institutions. The editors contacted the reviewers through their formal institutional affiliation and both reviewers denied knowledge of the manuscript. The editors then contacted the authors who reported that they had hired a company to assist with publishing. They paid the company RMB 3000 (equivalent to $430). The editors retracted the paper and contacted the Chinese Ministry of Science and Technology to investigate. Because of the fraud, the *British Journal of Clinical Pharmacology* analyzed and revised their entire peer review process.

IMPLICIT BIASES IN PEER REVIEW

Implicit biases are unconscious stereotypes that influence attitudes, behaviors, and beliefs toward other groups of people. In the United States, biases are often related to age, gender, weight, skin tone, or physical fitness and ability. Implicit biases may also be considered a form of confirmation bias. When someone fits the expected image of a banker, a teacher, or a coach, we tend to trust them, facilitating interactions. On the negative side, this trust makes us vulnerable to fraud. Scientists are often viewed as rational, intelligent, and dedicated professionals—and typically white males. Because of these biases, peers, journalists, and members of the public may either accept someone as an expert who is not or overlook actual experts.

Scientists have names for biases that exclude or dismiss the achievements of certain people. The *Matthew Effect* was coined by sociologist Robert Merton in a presentation to the American Sociological Association in 1968. Merton created the term based on the Gospel of Matthew, "To those who have, more will be given. From those who have little, even that will be taken from them." The Matthew Effect refers to how scientists, journalists, and members of the public disproportionately credit a preeminent scientist with a discovery. In a team of scientists, the well-known scientist is given primary credit. In many cases, collaborators are students who do most of the work and are unable to demand appropriate credit from senior scientists. Another form of Matthew Effect is when the discovery is made simultaneously by several scientists. The lesser-known scientist is overlooked in favor of the well-known scientist. For example, National Institutes of Health researcher Robert Gallo claimed credit for discovering the human immunodeficiency virus (HIV) in 1984. Gallo's virus was later identified as the exact same virus isolated by Luc Montagnier of the Pasteur Institute a year earlier. After years of dispute, the two scientists agreed to share credit. Allocation of credit is important because it increases the number of journal citations and impacts future funding. The more someone gets credit, the more research support they get, the more research they can do, and the more they get credit. Likewise, the scientist who is overlooked for credit must work harder for research funding. To game the system of credit, some scientists use Internet crawlers to pump up their number of citations. Merton's theory of Matthew Effect was developed from his wife's research, Harriet Zuckerman. Zuckerman studied the academic connections of 1966–1976 Nobel Prize winners and found that awardees who worked at the top 12 Nobel Prize winning institutions averaged 8.6 years of research before obtaining the award while those working elsewhere averaged 10.7 years of research before winning the Nobel Prize (Zuckerman 1967). On average, award winners working elsewhere were 10 years older than award winners at elite institutions.

Matilda Effect is when accomplishments by women are dismissed, minimized, or attributed to men. The problem is particularly strong in male-dominated disciplines including health and medicine. For example:

- Francis Crick, James Watson, and Maurice Wilkins won the Nobel Prize in Physiology and Medicine for the discovery of the double helix nature of DNA. Crick and Watson created their model based on Rosalind Franklin's work and images at King's College. When Franklin transferred from King's College to Birkbeck College, her colleagues/supervisors told her that King's College owned her images. She could not take her work to another institution. The colleagues then passed her images to Crick and Watson at Cambridge University!

- Nobel Prize–winning physicist Marie Curie was never awarded entry to the French Academy of Sciences.

- Esther Lederberg created the laboratory technique of transferring bacterial colonies from one petri dish to another. The technique allowed scientists to study antibiotic resistance. Her husband, Joshua Lederberg and coinvestigators George Beadle and Edward Tatum were awarded the Nobel Prize for the discovery.
- Nettie Stevens discovered that gender is determined by X-Y chromosomes. Thomas Hunt Morgan won the Nobel Prize for the achievement.

Taking credit for another person's work or refusing to give credit where credit is due are forms of scientific misconduct. The discredited person must work harder for funding and support. The additional effort wastes energy that could be applied to new investigations. Researchers at the University of Toronto analyzed 24,000 grant applications to the Canadian Institutes of Health Research and found that gender biases influenced grant reviews (Giannakeas, Sopik, and Narod 2019). When reviewers were asked to assess the application based on science, there was a gender gap of 0.9 percent. When reviewers were asked to assess the application based on leadership and expertise of the researcher, there was a gender gap of four percentage points. The researchers concluded that female scientists often contribute more labor for less credit.

Recent attention has turned toward the issue of *manels*, all male panels at conferences. Several prominent history and political science conferences failed to invite female speakers with the explanation that they did not know any female scholars. In response to manels, history scholars who identify as females started the #WOMENALSOKNOWHISTORY database to connect journalists, conference organizers, and editors with female historians. Political science scholars started the #WOMENALSOKNOWSTUFF database. In 2019, NIH director Francis Collins announced that in a personal effort toward greater inclusiveness in the STEM disciplines, he would no longer attend manels. While there has been greater awareness of exclusionary scholarship and taking credit for women's work, there is still much work to be done to eliminate implicit biases and create a fair system of credit and support.

REPLICATION OF STUDIES

Once study results are announced through conferences or journals, other researchers try to replicate the study results. In the best-case scenario, results are replicated before dissemination to popular news outlets. However, public demand for interesting news means that journalists are constantly scanning and searching for stories that will attract news customers. Releasing results before other scientists have an opportunity to respond to study findings is ill-advised. In 1979, epidemiologist Nancy Wertheimer and partner Ed Leeper published a study in which they investigated the theory that power lines cause childhood cancer. In a case-control study, Wertheimer visited the homes of Denver children with cancer. The couple compared neighborhood characteristics, traffic congestion, social class, and family structure to a control group. Study results found higher density of electrical wires in the neighborhoods of children with cancer. The researchers concluded that there may be a correlation between cancer and electromagnetic fields (Wertheimer and Leeper 1979). Although there were major methodological issues with how Wertheimer and Leeper selected their sample and measured electrical current, the study was published in the *American Journal of Epidemiology*. To measure electromagnetic fields, the couple did not take actual measurements. They estimated exposure based on thickness of electrical wires and proximity to the child's house. As other scientists attempted to replicate the findings using different methods, *New Yorker* journalist Paul Brodeur picked up the news story. A decade before the Wertheimer-Leeper study, Brodeur was instrumental in educating the public on the hazards of asbestos. He interviewed Dr. Irving Selikoff, reviewed records and provided evidence supporting the landmark lawsuit of Clarence Borel's estate (see chapter 4). Brodeur wrote a frightening three-part article on the Wertheimer-Leeper study and two subsequent books alleging that the power industry and the government were conspiring to cover up the link between childhood leukemia and power lines. Over the next few years, about 100 studies investigated the correlation between cancer and power lines. In 1996, the National Research Council announced that there was no consistent and conclusive evidence showing that exposure to residential electric or magnetic fields produced cancer or other adverse developmental effect (Committee on the Possible Effects of Electromagnetic Fields on Biologic Systems, Commission on Life Sciences, Division on Earth and Life Studies, and National Research Council 1997). Professor of Physics John W. Farley (2003) points out that the ongoing scare over power lines arises from the combination of three factors: a convincing author with a frightening story (Brodeur), a causal factor that most people do not understand and seems mysterious and threatening (electromagnetic fields), and a large for-profit company as the source of the problem (power companies). It can be difficult to differentiate public advocacy and scaremongering. Scientists need time to test the results of a study before final conclusions and policies can or should be determined.

YELLOW JOURNALISM

Yellow journalism is sleazy, sensational journalism designed to attract readers and increase circulation. The term developed in the late 1800s when William Randolph Hearst and Joseph Pulitzer competed for newspaper sales in New York City. Journalists for the two newspapers focused on sex, crime, deceit, and the dark sides of humanity. The newspapers printed headlines in large font with lots of pictures and images. Throughout history, reporters had always exaggerated a little. A good story sold more newspapers. Pulitzer created an empire on misleading stories. The standards of reporting lowered even further with William Randolph Hearst. Hearst was the only child of George Hearst, a poor prospector who struck it rich on the Comstock Lode, the first major silver discovery in the United States. George Hearst bought the *San Francisco Examiner* to further his political career. The newspaper advocated for Hearst to become U.S. senator for California. The Hearst's doted on their son. William was arrogant and spoiled. He was expelled from Harvard for multiple pranks the most notable of which was sending chamber pots to his professors. Each chamber pot had an image of the professor printed inside.

Young Hearst was attracted to journalism and spent a short time working at Pulitzer's New York newspaper, the *New York World*. In 1887, Hearst took over his father's newspaper. With vast wealth to support his interest, he purchased the latest equipment and hired the best journalists. For several years, the *Examiner* lost money. However, Hearst knew his readers and modeled his business on Pulitzer's eccentric style. Hearst saw himself as a champion of the poor and disenfranchised. His journalists created excitement and human interest even when there was none. The *Examiner* focused on social issues, such as exposing low standards of treatment in the city's hospital or horrific working conditions in the cannery business. The newspaper frequently criticized the monopoly of California's Southern Pacific Railroad. Before long, the newspaper enjoyed the largest circulation of any San Francisco newspaper and started making a lot of money through advertising.

In 1895, Hearst expanded his empire by purchasing the *New York Morning Journal*. He immediately began hiring journalists and artists away from the *World*. Some left for better pay while others left because Pulitzer was demanding and temperamental. In comparison, Hearst treated his staff very well. Pulitzer fought back. Hearst stepped up his marketing with posters, brass bands, and free coffee for customers. He reduced the price of the *Morning Journal* from two cents to a penny. One very popular comic strip of the time was *Hogan's Alley*. The cartoon appeared in the *World*. It featured life in New York City's tenement slums through the experiences and thoughts of a hairless (probably due to lice), barefoot little boy in a large yellow nightshirt. The Yellow Kid was one of very few comics that contained color. The yellow nightshirt represented the faded hand-me-down clothing of many poor families. Hearst hired the Yellow Kid creator, Richard F. Outcault away from the *World*. In response, the *World* hired a second artist, George Luks, to draw the Yellow Kid. Two artists were drawing the same political commentary comic in two different newspapers at the same time. As Hearst and Pulitzer competed for readership and advertising, the newspapers degenerated into sensationalism and the term *yellow journalism* arose.

The power of yellow journalism could not be underestimated. Hearst regularly published stories reporting conflicts between a large, oppressive force and a poor, oppressed group of people. The stories did not only increase readership, they forged people together and created a brand. One regular target was the Spanish government in Cuba. The *Morning Journal* presented the Cuban people as noble resistors of a cruel oppressive Spanish government. The publishers knew that a war would increase newspaper circulation. While both New York newspapers prodded for war, both countries resisted. Neither government wanted to go to war. On February 15, 1898, the USS *Maine* exploded in Havana Harbor. Two hundred and sixty people died. Although the cause of the explosion was unknown, Hearst immediately published a conspiracy theory accusing pro-Spanish sympathizers. Both Hearst and Pulitzer rallied the public and instigated the Spanish-American War of 1898.

Although yellow journalism enjoyed wide readership, the journalists, newspapers, and businessmen were not respected. Pulitzer eventually backed off sensational reporting and became known for journalistic integrity. Hearst continued the practice. In 1901, two journalists published separate articles suggesting that Hearst's yellow journalism had driven Leon Czolgosz to assassinate President William McKinley. Hearst's reputation never recovered from the accusation. Today, yellow journalism appears as scaremongering headlines, misleading content, mismatched headlines and content, pseudoscience, faked interviews, or manipulated images. Authors present themselves as experts even though they have little to no knowledge on the topic. For example, Nina Teicholz is an investigative journalist who earned a master's degree in Latin American studies. Without any background in biology or nutrition, Teicholz published a book questioning the nutritional advice to limit intake of saturated fats. Teicholz advises readers to eat butter and drink whole milk. Despite criticism by leading experts, the book made the *New York Times* best-seller list, the *Wall Street Journal* top 10 nonfiction books, and *The Economist* best science books. Beef industry leaders applaud Teicholz for advocating diets rich in animal fats and protein. Meanwhile over 645,000 people die each year due to heart disease.

The 24-hour news cycle and cable news immunizes readers and viewers to accept yellow journalism. With constant access to news, consumers want new and exciting stories. If a media outlet is not reporting new news, the consumer moves to another outlet. Facts become secondary to entertainment. Journalists compete for stories and will skip over details in a hurried effort to get the story into the news as quickly as possible. In a rush to publish, journalists do not check facts, verify stories, or provide relevance. For example, consider the news of a study by National Institutes of Health researchers suggesting that coffee drinkers live longer (Freedman et al. 2012). The study surveyed over 400,000 people and calculated a modest inverse association between coffee drinking and total mortality. Since coffee is one of the most widely consumed beverages in the world, the news is of interest to many readers. Of the dozens of media outlets that carried the story, most failed to mention that the study also found that coffee drinkers were more likely to smoke cigarettes, drink three alcoholic beverages per day, eat more red meat and less fresh fruits and vegetables, engage in less vigorous physical activity, and have lower education levels. These are all risk factors for chronic disease. The researchers only found the association after they made statistical adjustments for the major risk factors. Furthermore, the relationship was an association not causal (see chapter 4). News reports neglected to mention the link between drinking coffee and smoking or the fact that what someone puts in their coffee (sugar or cream) also influences longevity. Another misleading technique of journalists is pseudosymmetry. Pseudosymmetry presents two individuals facing off in debate over an issue. This technique is commonly used in climate change debates with one scientist warning of climate change while the other refutes climate change. In reality, 99 percent of scientists agree that climate change exists while only 1 percent deny the phenomenon. Pseudosymmetry misleads viewers into thinking that an issue is more controversial or questionable than it actually is. A final mechanism to hook readers is conspiracy theories. People, regardless of education, are fascinated by conspiracy theories. Conspiracy theories surrounding the Sandy Hook elementary school shooting, pizzagate, vaccinations, and many other issues are constantly creating fear and suspicion. The 24-hour news cycle influences consumer demand and consumer demand influences journalistic standards of the 24-hour news cycle.

DEMO DOLLIES AND PUBLICITY HOUNDS

Demo dollies are the men and women hired at trade shows to sell a product. The main criterion for the job is physical attractiveness. There is no requirement to actually know how the product works or to understand the technology behind the product. Elizabeth Holmes (chapter 1) is a good example of a demo dolly. The young, pretty, blond-haired woman presented herself as a business magnate and created an impressive front cover for many popular magazines. When journalists, talk show hosts, or news shows are looking for stories, they also want people who will attract attention, people who are handsome or pretty, trendy, and charismatic. They want demo dollies. Damian Jacob Markiewicz Sendler (aka Damian Dariusz Markiewicz) was one such character. Sendler was the perfect interviewee. The confident, handsome young man reported extremely impressive credentials: a master's degree, MD, and PhD in sexual behavior from Harvard University, one of the youngest members in the American Psychiatric Association and the American Academy of Psychiatry and the Law, awarded the U.S. President's Gold Service Award for humanitarian work, and chief of sexology at a nonprofit research institute. Sendler published multiple research articles on necrophilia, zoophilia, erotic asphyxiation, and sexual assault. He was quoted by *Playboy*, *Huffington Post*, *Women's Health*, *Forbes*, and many other popular adult magazines. He even offered online sex therapy until senior editor and reporter at Gizmodo, Jennings Brown decided to check out Sendler's background. There was no record of Sendler earning an MD or PhD. Sendler was enrolled in Harvard's Extension School as a master's candidate. Harvard does not offer a PhD in sexual behavior. There is no Gold Service award for humanitarian work by the U.S. president. Sendler was a student member of the American Academy of Psychiatry and the Law and although he did manage a website describing a research institute with the names of 28 staff, Brown could find no evidence that any of the colleagues existed. Sendler did successfully publish research articles. Most of his studies were case studies. With greater context, Brown wondered whether the cases even existed. In articles and interviews, Sendler consistently used insensitive language, language strongly discouraged by experts in the field. When Brown inquired about Sendler's credentials, Sendler responded by claiming that he had told Harvard not to release his academic qualifications. As Brown pushed further, Sendler responded that false qualifications are subjective because everyone misrepresents credentials and accomplishments to some degree.

Humans are naturally drawn to attractive, confident, gregarious, and charismatic people. This attraction may be inherent. In past civilizations, survival depended on having a leader who could mobilize community members to collect food, provide safety, and care for the young. People with magnetic personalities, with lots of charisma, are able to bypass naysayers and rally the group toward a mission. Charismatic leaders allow communities to survive and thrive. The *Doctor Fox Effect* describes how even the most educated people are taken in by charismatic speakers. The Dr. Fox Effect is based on a study at University of California School of Medicine in which three groups of psychiatrists, psychologists, social work academics, and educational administrators attended a lecture by "Dr. Myron Fox" of Albert Einstein College of Medicine (Naftulin, Ware, and Donnelly 1973). The speaker bio noted that Dr. Fox had written two books and several articles on the application of mathematics to human behavior. Dr. Fox was actually actor Michael Fox who was coached to deliver an expressive and engaging lecture filled with double talk, illogical statements, and invented words. In the speaker evaluation, attendees rated the actor very highly. Although the original study is criticized for lack of a control group, replications indicate that regardless of competency, engaging speakers consistently rank higher than unengaging speakers. In his book, *Why Do So Many Incompetent Men Become Leaders? (And How to Fix It)*, Tomas Chamorro-Premuzic explains that the problem with preference for charismatic leaders is that it causes people to overlook potential warning signs. Charismatic leaders tend to ignore or deny obstacles or bad news in order to maintain support and positive attitudes. They offer unrealistic solutions to complex problems, which ultimately puts the community at risk of failure. Appearing in the news or receiving massive public attention can be thrilling for some people. Publicity hounds are people who will do anything for media attention, including antagonizing people.

Ward LeRoy Churchill

Ward LeRoy Churchill earned an MA in Communications Theory from Sangamon State University, now University of Illinois, Springfield. Within a few years of graduation, he worked as an administrator and part-time lecturer in American Indian Studies, Film Studies, and Sociology at the University of Colorado Boulder. The scholar-activist wrote over a dozen books, 20 journal articles, and 70 essays challenging popular beliefs. He gained notoriety through controversy. His ideas on the Holocaust, racism, feminism, and Native Americans drew both praise and rebuke. In 1990, University of Colorado Boulder offered Churchill a full-time faculty position in the Department of Ethnic Studies. Within a year, he was given tenure, a process that normally takes six years. In 2005, Churchill wrote *On the Justice of Roosting Chickens* in which he declared that the September 11, 2001, attacks were the result of U.S. involvement in the Middle East. Churchill described the people working in the World Trade Center as "a technocratic corps at the very heart of America's global financial empire" and "little Eichmanns," a reference to the Holocaust. In 1996, Professor John P. LaVelle raised concerns that Churchill deliberately misrepresented information from the General Allotment Act of 1887 (an act to divide Native American lands by the federal government). The University of Colorado investigated Churchill on seven allegations of fabrication, falsification, and plagiarism and found evidence supporting six of the allegations. In concluding statements, the investigative report noted:

> We believe that the University of Colorado may have made the extraordinary decision to hire Professor Churchill, a charismatic public intellectual with no doctorate and no history of regular faculty membership at a university, to a tenured position without any probationary period in part because at that moment in the institution's history, it desired the favorable attention his notoriety and following were expected to bring. . . . The university has perhaps gotten more than it bargained for when it made its high-risk decisions about Professor Churchill . . . the indignation now exhibited by some University actors about Churchill's work appears disingenuous, as they and their predecessors are the ones who decided to hire him. (Wesson et al. 2006, 100)

Churchill blamed his editor, his publisher, his assistant, his former spouse, and a collaborator for the scholarly misconduct. The committee was split on whether to terminate Churchill. The university did subsequently fire him. He sued the university for wrongful termination and was awarded $1 million. The award was later overturned by the district court. As the investigators noted, Churchill did not have the knowledge or the training to engage in responsible scholarship. He chased fame by skipping over facts.

DISINFORMATION

Disinformation is false information, intended to mislead or deceive people. Disinformation is often rooted in a political or financial agenda. Organizer of the Boston Tea Party, Sam Adams, stoked anti-British sentiment by regularly publishing articles in the *Journal of Occurrences* (Streitmatter 2012). Adams reported profane and abusive behavior by British soldiers with stories of drunkenness, rape, and assault against the people of Boston. Adams did not name the accusers or the accused. The victims were typically described as good, law-abiding citizens while the British soldiers were described as evil villains. Although British officials denied the accusations, Adams's sensational reports became very popular. Within six months, hostility against British troops grew to such a point that the British withdrew four regiments of militiamen from Boston. Adams continued his media campaign by tacking fliers on trees and tavern doors during the night. Disinformation spreads quickly and is difficult to deconstruct once it is out there. Modern examples of disinformation include Andrew Wakefield's claim that vaccinations cause autism, anti-abortionists' claims that abortion causes breast cancer, and the idea that HIV was created by the CIA.

AIDS Disinformation

In 1979, Russia invaded Afghanistan. U.S. president Ronald Reagan responded by suspending arms reduction talks and increasing military spending. In 1982, Yuri Andropov was elected general-secretary of the Communist Party. The former KGB chairman was highly intelligent, patient, and calm. He also liked conspiracy theories, a trait that may have been heightened by electrolyte imbalances due to chronic kidney disease. On July 17, 1983, an obscure newspaper in India, the *Patriot*, published the headlines, "AIDS may invade India: Mystery disease caused by US experiments." The *Patriot* was founded in 1967 with the help of the KGB. The paper was known for featuring Soviet-related articles. The article relied on an anonymous letter written by a "well-known American scientist and anthropologist" in New York. Comingling fact and fiction, the letter cited publicly available government information while also claiming that AIDS was discovered at Fort Detrick, Maryland, through CIA-sponsored biological weapons testing. The author alleged that the U.S. government was planning to transfer the experiments to Pakistan, threatening public health in Pakistan and India. The assertion reflected earlier claims in the Soviet media reporting that Lahore, Pakistan, was a biological warfare facility managed by U.S. scientists. The letter contained other information suggesting that the source was not a "well-known American scientist and anthropologist" but actually the KGB. The article went unnoticed until 1985 when fears of AIDS grew and the U.S. government claimed that the Soviets were producing biological weapons. The Soviet press published an article again mixing fact and story and referencing the *Patriot* article.

Jakob Segal was a well-respected East German biophysicist, retired and living in France. Segal and his wife were empathetic of those suffering from AIDS and supportive of the Soviet bloc. Segal started publishing pamphlets refuting that the virus originated in Africa. His premise was that AIDS was first identified among gay men in New York and San Francisco. Segal believed that the U.S. government infected male prisoners who then infected other men. Segal believed that if Americans believed that their government created AIDS, people would lose faith in the government. He attacked fellow East German scientists who contested his theory by accusing them of conspiring with the U.S. government. The U.S. government was aware of what was going on. The Active Measures Working Group (AMWG) was created in 1981 to monitor and counter Soviet-sponsored disinformation campaigns. The State Department pointed out that Segal's explanation of how AIDS was created did not match basic biological techniques and that AIDS had been documented as early as 1959. As the number of AIDS cases increased in Moscow, it became apparent that scientists needed to work with one another. The Soviet Academy of Sciences refuted the idea that AIDS was created in a laboratory. However, Segal maintained his theory until death in 1995 and the theory continues to grow long after his death. In Zimbabwe, a letter to the editor accused the U.S. of exporting AIDS-contaminated condoms to foreign countries. Nobel Peace Prize winner Wangari Maathai claimed that the disease was created to eliminate people of color. A 2005 study found that an estimated 50 percent of African Americans believed that AIDS was manmade (Bogart and Thorburn 2005). In reviewing AIDS disinformation, senior historian at the U.S. Army Center of Military History, Thomas Boghardt reports that the techniques used to create and spread disinformation were simple consisting of: scapegoating, constant repetition, and mixing of facts and fabrication. The problem is that deliberate misinformation is difficult to counter and remove from public record and public opinion.

ANTI-INTELLECTUALISM

Anti-intellectualism is antipathy toward educated people. Characteristics of anti-intellectualism are contempt for education, distrust of science, and the perception that scholars are arrogant and out of touch with the real world. Anti-intellectuals view themselves as working people with common sense whose thoughts and ideas are belittled and dismissed by the political and academic elite. The ideology is also a technique of dictators and fascist governments to control information and suppress political dissent. By disparaging intellectuals, totalitarian governments isolate and silence those who might question them. Military, pseudo-military, cults, and fundamental religious groups encourage anti-intellectual thought as a way to control beliefs and behaviors. The ideology forges cohesion through an *us against them* attitude.

The dismissal of science in favor of personal ideas and philosophies hinders social progress. For example, rather than investigating and using an evidence-based bullying prevention intervention, anti-intellectuals may use what they believe works, such as peer mediation. Peer mediation is not an effective form of bullying intervention because peers are easily drawn into supporting the charming and likeable bully, blaming the victim for the abuse. Anti-intellectualism can cause significant harm. Anti-intellectual ideology allows fraudsters to take advantage of people. The basic tenet of the philosophy favors expediency over critical thinking. For example, Elizabeth Holmes and Sunny Balwani presented Holmes as a biotech genius who invented a machine to test blood chemistry despite the fact that she had no education in the field (see chapter 1). Investors, journalists, magazine editors, talk show hosts, and company leaders fell for the fairy tale. They wanted to believe that someone could succeed without education or training. The problem is that expediency encourages cheating. For those without internal moral controls, it is easier to lie and cheat than to do the hard work required to learn engineering, biology, or medicine. A college degree is seen as a tool for money rather than an opportunity to cultivate critical thinking.

Anti-intellectualism exists on a scale. Behaviors range from the illusion of explanatory depth to confirmation bias to vicious attacks on scientists and scholars. The illusion of explanatory depth (IOED) is a concept where people believe they know more than they actually do (Rozenblit and Keil 2002). IOED relates to common, everyday tools, occurrences, or theories. The person suffering from IOED may have pieces of understanding yet lacks depth and full understanding. In one study of IOED, Dr. Rebecca Lawson (2006) of the University of Liverpool asked 81 study volunteers to sketch a bicycle. Most of the participants knew how to ride a bicycle and at least half owned a bicycle. The sketches revealed multiple errors such as placing the pedals on the front wheel or drawing the angle of the handlebars where they could not possibly turn the wheel. When shown a functioning bicycle, many volunteers were surprised by their errors. The illusion of explanatory depth is a deception. When people see, use, or experience objects every day, they assume that they know and understand the item more than they actually do. Because of the IOED, people dismiss information that might take them to deeper level of understanding.

Confirmation bias was described from the standpoint of data collection in chapter 6. The concept also applies to nonscientists. With confirmation bias, people will embrace ideas that support their beliefs and reject ideas that counter their beliefs. Denialism of climate change is an example of confirmation bias. Despite verifiable studies showing global warming, many politicians, religious leaders, and corporations denounce the problem. In *Denying to the Grave: Why We Ignore the Facts That Will Save Us*, Drs. Sara and Jack Gorman explore why people refuse to vaccinate their children, believe that a gun will protect them from violence, and do not trust genetically modified foods. Researchers at Brown University found that confirmation bias varied by genetics (Doll, Hutchison, and Frank 2011). Polymorphism of the *COMT* gene (rs4680) was predictive of the degree of confirmation bias. Experts believe that when someone reads or perceives information that supports current beliefs, the neurotransmitter dopamine is released in the body. One function of dopamine in the body involves reward-motivated behavior. Dopamine signals desirability or aversion to an experience. If someone reads information confirming beliefs, they experience positive feelings or cognitive similarity. If they read something counter to current beliefs, they experience negative feelings or cognitive dissonance. People prefer cognitive similarity. They will dismiss information that creates cognitive dissonance (Mercier and Sperber 2017).

CENSORSHIP

Throughout history, many authoritarian governments, religious institutions, businesses, and organizations have attempted to control knowledge by censoring those with differing opinions. Censorship is the suppression of speech or information. Reasons for censorship include concerns that obscene or objectionable material will corrupt society or threaten public safety. Books, movies, songs, even research may be censored. The criterion for censorship is in the eyes of the beholder. In Nazi Germany, an estimated 20,000 books written by Jewish, communist, or humanist authors were burned on funeral pyres. Newspapers, radio stations, and book publishers were taken over to control information and disseminate Nazi propaganda. The German government shut down media agencies that refused to cooperate. During Apartheid, the South African government censored music, clothing, and literature. The Publications Act of 1974 forbid any expression considered "blasphemous, or . . . offensive to the religious convictions or feelings of any section of the inhabitants of the Republic." Banned items included the music record *Hair*, T-shirts with "Black is Beautiful," any buttons, badges, or T-shirts with symbols of the African National Conference (ANC) as well as books by William Faulkner, Tennessee Williams, and Angela Davis. Censorship allows those in power to maintain power by controlling knowledge, communication, and potential dissent. Those who speak out or violate censorship laws face retaliation, job dismissal, blacklisting, violence, imprisonment, or exile. Suppression is a path to oppression, the persecution or abuse of certain people. In her keynote address to the 2018 Scholars at Risk Global Congress, Dr. Judith Butler referred to the oppression of science as the criminalization of knowledge. Historically, when authorities attempt to control information, it doesn't work. Knowledge does not go away. It is driven underground fostering a counterculture that, with enough support, will swell, rebel, and overcome suppression.

Suppression of information stymies health and social advances. In the 1990s, the National Rifle Association (NRA) lobbied Congress to pass the Dickey Amendment banning the allocation of federal funds for research that could suggest the need for gun control. The NRA wanted to stop a developing line of research showing that guns in the home were more likely to injure someone living in the home than a home invader. Although multiple professional health and medical organizations objected to the amendment and requested repeal, the federal government stood by the ban. In 2012, the murder of 20 six- and seven-year-old children and six adults at Sandy Hook Elementary School spurred demand for action. While the shootings in Newtown, Connecticut, was the impetus for change, Sandy Hook was one in a long history of school shootings. Between September 30, 1996, when the Dickey Amendment passed and December 14, 2012, the date of the Sandy Hook Elementary School shooting, there were 114 school shootings. Two hundred and five people, mostly children, were killed and 276 people were physically injured. The emotional and mental injury is beyond measurement. While children were being shot in schools, researchers struggled to get funding for gun violence research. Many times, researchers can turn to other countries to catch up on lost time. In this case, no other country has the type of gun laws that the United States has. The culture limits benchmarking to other areas.

In addition to politics, corporations may attempt to silence researchers. In the early 1980s, Victor DeNoble and Paul Mele were researchers at Philip Morris, investigating a substitute for nicotine that did not cause heart attack and stroke. The researchers discovered a substitute. The substance was highly addictive and required FDA oversight. In 1983, DeNoble and coauthors wrote a manuscript on nicotine addiction. Philip Morris lawyers forced the researchers to withdraw the manuscript because it provided legal evidence of physical and behavioral addiction to cigarettes. In 1984, DeNoble and Mele were fired. In order to receive severance packages, they were required to sign confidentiality agreements promising to never discuss their research. In 1994, Congress was investigating the effects of cigarette smoking and asked DeNoble and Mele to give testimony about their research. Both men initially refused citing the nondisclosure agreement. Congress pressured Philip Morris to drop the restriction and both men testified to the fact that Philip Morris knew and tried to hide evidence regarding the addictive nature of cigarettes.

Since people do not like change or to have their existing ideas challenged, scholars often experience threats or retaliation. The organization, Scholars at

Risk reports and maps more than 300 cases per year of scholars who have been threatened with execution, imprisonment, or job termination as the result of politically charged questions or ideas. One of the cases is that of Pinar Selek. Selek is a sociologist who documented the suppression and oppression of lesbian, gay, bisexual, and transgender individuals and Kurdish communities in Turkey. The Kurds are a minority population who have suffered forced inscription, forced relocation, mass arrest, imprisonment, torture, and execution at the hands of Turkish authorities. The European Court of Human Rights named Turkey the leading violator of the European Convention of Human Rights in 2011. Since 1984, the terrorist organization, the Kurdistan Workers' Party (PKK) has led attacks on Turkish authorities and villages. The PKK has also been criticized for human rights violations, abduction of children for training as soldiers, the use of suicide bombers, and drug trafficking. Selek wrote extensively on human rights issues in Turkey and founded a magazine focused on feminist concerns. On July 9, 1998, there was an explosion in the Istanbul Spice Bazaar. Seven people died and 127 were wounded. Selek was working on a street art project when she was arrested and charged with bombing the market. A codefendant, Abdülmecit Öztürk was also arrested and charged. During interrogation, Öztürk implicated Selek. He later recanted his testimony in court. Selek served two and a half years in jail. She reported being tortured and pressured to make a false confession. In 2000, experts determined that the explosion was caused by a gas leak. Selek was released and rearrested in 2005. She was subjected to a new trial related to the explosion and eventually acquitted. When the acquittal was reversed, Selek fled to France. In 2012, Selek was charged again. The court found her guilty in 2013. In 2014, Selek's conviction was overturned on procedural grounds. The charges remained intact. Selek was retried in 2014 and acquitted. The time and effort to attend to legal accusations interfered with her scholarly productivity. Selek maintains that the court cases are the result of her research including connections with members of PKK. Scholars at Risk recognizes the obligation of countries to maintain public safety while also honoring academic freedom and due process.

Censorship may actually be a reasonable solution for some research topics. In 2002, researchers from the State University of New York at Stony Brook published a paper in *Science* describing synthesis of live polio virus from HeLa cells (Cello, Aniko, and Wimmer 2002). Readers raised concerns that the description of study procedures could be used by bioterrorists to create the virus and stage an attack. Other researchers published a study in the *Journal of Urology* reporting successful engineering of mouse pox virus. Given concerns over the potential for laboratory synthesis of lethal pathogens, the scientists chose to self-censure their own research. Censorship may be an option in cases where the knowledge does not advance society and instead has the potential to harm people.

ACADEMIC FREEDOM

To ensure that research is not censured by politics, religion, corporate interest, or society, colleges and universities are bound by the concept of academic freedom. Academic freedom is freedom of scholars to research, discuss, and disseminate information that may be unpopular or uncomfortable. Institutions of higher education cannot fire a professor for *professing* the truth. Academic freedom allows scholars to raise challenging questions in order to advance society. For example, after training as a psychiatrist at Harvard Medical School, Morris E. Chafetz reluctantly took a job starting an alcohol treatment center. No one else wanted the job, and it was the only one he could get. Chafetz did not like alcoholics. Like many others, he viewed alcoholism as a moral weakness. After a few months in clinical practice, he realized that his patients were people with a disease just like any other disease. He lobbied for a government agency to address the issue of alcoholism and became the first director of the National Institute on Alcohol Abuse and Alcoholism. Chafetz used initial funding to educate society about alcoholism, treatment, and support. He later went on to work at Johns Hopkins University as a research scientist. Despite highly controversial views, such as teaching elementary school children responsible drinking, Chafetz was able to change attitudes towards alcoholism in order to improve treatment and prevention of the disorder.

Although academic institutions promise academic freedom, there have been cases where money trumps academic freedom. In 1990, Betty C. Dong and colleagues at UC San Francisco concluded a study finding that generic forms of levothyroxine, a drug used to treat hypothyroidism, were just as effective as the name brand drug, Synthroid. The research was funded by Boots Pharmaceuticals Inc. Boots objected to the study results and suppressed publication by invoking a contractual clause on publications. The company and the researchers debated publication for four years. The university hired independent peer reviewers who provided positive feedback on the research while a Boots-funded researcher and journal editor ripped the study apart. Dong submitted the manuscript for publication and Boots executives threatened to sue her. The university notified her that they would not defend her if she proceeded with publication. Under pressure from the FDA, the university reluctantly agreed not to block publication. It took seven years for the research to get published. The delay is estimated to have cost consumers using the name brand drug over $2 billion (Maugh 1997).

There are limits to academic freedom. James Frederick Tracy was a tenured associate professor in the School of Communication and Multimedia Studies, Florida Atlantic University. He maintained a personal blog that espoused conspiracy theories. In 2013, Tracy used his personal blog to endorse the opinion that the Sandy Hook shooting was a staged hoax, an attempt to push for gun control. Tracy's "evidence" was that media reports were missing pictures of the victims' bodies and emergency medical care professionals at work. Tracy also advertised his book, *Nobody Died at Sandy Hook* on his blog. Florida Atlantic University reprimanded Tracy on the grounds that he did not make it clear that he was not speaking on behalf of the college. Tracy continued his agenda, sending a certified letter to grieving parents Lenny and Veronique Pozner. The Pozners were still reeling from the loss of their six-year-old son, Noah, when Tracy demanded proof of their son's existence. Noah's funeral was the first funeral of Sandy Hook victims. Mrs. Pozner insisted on an open casket so that the world could see what the attacker had done to the little boy in a batman shirt and Spider-Man sneakers. Conspiracy theorists inundated the Pozners with death threats, demands to exhume their son's body, and horrible accusations. The Pozners asked Florida Atlantic to terminate Tracy for giving academic credence to the lies and attacks. Tracy defended his statements as a search for the truth and claimed his termination was retaliation for speaking out. The purpose of academic freedom is to embolden researchers to study new and amazing topics without fear of retaliation. Academic freedom does not give someone the right to intentionally harm another person.

Researchers are judged on the quality of their research, the number of publications, and the quality of the venue where articles are published. The pressure to publish or perish while still engaging in time-intensive research means that some people are tempted to take short cuts. While ideally, new discoveries and research findings should be released as soon as possible, there are benefits to going through the slow and deliberate process of peer review. Bypassing peer review and disseminating information directly to popular media creates confusion and opportunity for less credible sources to emerge. There is also a need for journalists to check sources, verify information and report subtle details of a new study finding.

FURTHER READING

Bogart, Laura M., and Sheryl Thorburn. 2005. "Are HIV/AIDS Conspiracy Beliefs a Barrier to HIV Prevention among African Americans?" *Journal of Acquired Immune Deficiency Syndromes* 38 (2): 213–18.

Boghardt, Thomas. 2009. "Soviet Bloc Intelligence and Its AIDS Disinformation Campaign." *Studies in Intelligence* 53 (4): 1–24. Accessed August 21, 2019. https://www.cia.gov/library/center-for-the-study-of-intelligence/csi -publications/csi-studies/studies/vol53no4/pdf/U-%20Boghardt-AIDS -Made%20in%20the%20USA-17Dec.pdf

Brown, Jennings. "The Fake Sex Doctor Who Conned the Media into Publicizing His Bizarre Research." Accessed November 19, 2019. https://gizmodo

.com/the-fake-sex-doctor-who-conned-the-media-into-publicizi
-1832711205

Cello, Jeronimo, Aniko V. Paul, and Eckard Wimmer. 2002. "Chemical Synthesis of Poliovirus CDNA: Generation of Infectious Virus in the Absence
of Natural Template." *Science* 297 (5583): 1016–18.

Chamorro-Premuzic, Tomas. 2019. *Why Do So Many Incompetent Men Become
Leaders?: (And How to Fix It).* Boston: Harvard Business School Press
Books.

Cohen, Adam, Smita Pattanaik, Praveen Kumar, Robert R. Bies, Anthonius Boer,
Albert Ferro, Annette Gilchrist, Geoffrey K. Isbister, Sarah Ross, and
Andrew J. Webb. 2016. "Organised Crime against the Academic Peer
Review System." *British Journal of Clinical Pharmacology* 81 (6):
1012–17.

Cohen, Daniel. 2000. "The Yellow Kid." In *Yellow Journalism*, 20. Minneapolis:
Lerner Publishing Group.

Committee on the Possible Effects of Electromagnetic Fields on Biologic Systems, Commission on Life Sciences, Division on Earth and Life Studies,
and National Research Council. 1997. "Possible Health Effects of Exposure to Residential Electric and Magnetic Fields." Washington, D.C.:
National Academies Press.

Doll, Bradley B., Kent E. Hutchison, and Michael J. Frank. 2011. "Dopaminergic
Genes Predict Individual Differences in Susceptibility to Confirmation
Bias." *Journal of Neuroscience* 31 (16): 6188–98.

Farley, John W. 2003. "Power Lines and Cancer: Nothing to Fear." Quachwatch
.org. Accessed August 21, 2019. https://www.quackwatch.org/01Quackery
RelatedTopics/emf.html

Freedman, Neal D., Yikyung Park, Christian C. Abnet, Rashmi Sinha, and Albert
R. Hollenbeck. 2012. "Association of Coffee Drinking with Total and
Cause-Specific Mortality." *New England Journal of Medicine* 366 (20):
1891–904.

Geissler, Erhard, and Robert Hunt Sprinkle. 2019. "Were Our Critics Right about
the Stasi?: AIDS Disinformation and 'Disinformation Squared' after
Five Years." *Politics & the Life Sciences* 38 (1): 32–61.

Giannakeas, Vasily, Victoria Sopik, and Steven Narod. 2019. "Gender Bias in
CIHR Foundation Grant Awarding." *Lancet* 393 (10187): 2195–2195.

Gliboff, Sander. 2018. "Sex and the Scientific Author: M. Vaerting and the
Matilda Effect in Early Twentieth-Century Germany." *Gender & History*
30 (2): 490–510.

Godlee, Fiona, C. R. Gale, and C. N. Martyn. 1998. "Effect on the Quality of
Peer Review of Blinding Reviewers and Asking Them to Sign Their
Reports: A Randomized Controlled Trial." *JAMA* 280 (3): 237–40.

Gorman, Sara E, and Jack M. Gorman. 2017. *Denying to the Grave: Why We Ignore the Facts That Will Save Us.* New York: Oxford University Press.

Grabo, Allen, Brian R. Spisak, and Mark van Vugt. 2017. "Charisma as Signal: An Evolutionary Perspective on Charismatic Leadership." *Leadership Quarterly* 28 (4): 473–85.

Knobloch-Westerwick, Silvia, and Carroll J. Glynn. 2013. "The Matilda Effect—Role Congruity Effects on Scholarly Communication: A Citation Analysis of Communication Research and Journal of Communication Articles." *Communication Research* 40 (1): 3–26.

Knobloch-Westerwick, Silvia, and Caterina Keplinger. 2007. "Thrilling News: Factors Generating Suspense during News Exposure." *Media Psychology* 9 (1): 193–210.

Kolbert, Elizaveth. 2017. "That's What You Think." *New Yorker* 93 (2): 66–71.

Konnikova, Maria. 2017. *The Confidence Game: Why We Fall for It . . . Every Time.* London: Penguin Books.

Lawson, Rebecca. 2006. "The Science of Cycology: Failures to Understand How Everyday Objects Work." *Memory & Cognition* 34 (8): 1667–75.

Maugh, Thomas H. 1997. "Drug Firm Suppressed Test Data for Years, Doctors Say." *Los Angeles Times—Southern California Edition*, April 16. Accessed August 28, 2019. https://www.latimes.com/archives/la-xpm-1997-04-16-mn-49174-story.html

Mazur, Allan. 1989. "Biomedical Science in Supermarket Tabloids." *Knowledge, Technology & Policy* 2 (3): 74–81.

McDonald, Peter D. 2009. *The Literature Police: Apartheid Censorship and Its Cultural Consequences.* Oxford: Oxford University Press.

Mercier, Hugo, and Dan Sperber. 2017. *The Enigma of Reason.* Cambridge, MA: Harvard University Press.

Merton, Robert K. 1968. "The Matthew Effect in Science." *Science* 159 (3810): 56–63.

Naftulin, D. H., John E. Ware Jr., and F. A. Donnelly. 1973. "The Doctor Fox Lecture." *Journal of Medical Education* 48 (7): 630–35.

Rozenblit, Leonid, and Frank Keil. 2002. "The Misunderstood Limits of Folk Science: An Illusion of Explanatory Depth." *Cognitive Science* 26 (5): 521–62.

Smith, Richard. 1997. "Peer Review: Reform or Revolution? Time to Open up the Black Box of Peer Review." *British Medical Journal* 315 (7111): 759–60.

Spinner, Jenny. (2019). Personal Interview.

Streitmatter, Rodger. 2012. *Mightier Than the Sword: How the News Media Have Shaped American History.* 3rd ed. Boulder, CO: Westview Press.

Wahowiak, Lindsey. 2018. "Facts Not Enough: Public Health Working to Fight Misinformation through Trust, Relationships." *Nation's Health* 48 (5): 1–20.

Welsh, Jennifer. 2010. "Year's Best Peer Review Comments: Papers That 'Suck the Will to Live.'" *Discover.* Accessed August 28, 2019. http://blogs .discovermagazine.com/discoblog/2010/12/15/years-best-peer-review -comments-papers-that-suck-the-will-to-live/#.XULxfMQpBPY
Wertheimer, N., and E. Leeper. 1979. "Electrical Wiring Configurations and Childhood Cancer." *American Journal of Epidemiology* 109 (3): 273–84.
Wesson, Marianne, Robert N. Clinton, José E. Limón, Marjorie K. McIntosh, Michael L. Radalet, Linda Morris, and J. Eric Elliff. 2006. "Report of the Investigative Committee of the Standing Committee on Research Misconduct at the University of Colorado at Boulder concerning Allegations of Academic Misconduct against Professor Ward Churchill." Accessed August 28, 2019. https://web.archive.org/web/20060523111342/http:// www.colorado.edu/news/reports/churchill/download/WardChurchill Report.pdf
Zuckerman, H. 1967. "The Sociology of the Nobel Prizes." *Scientific American* 217 (5): 25–33.

NINE

Solutions

Medical research is both collaborative and competitive. Scientists must work with study participants, laboratory colleagues, other experts in the field, key stakeholders in the community, and journalists to advance humanity. Under the current systems, scientists must also compete for funding, laboratory space, jobs, and publications. To gain advantage, some people will try to take shortcuts or engage in misconduct. In a survey of National Institutes of Health researchers, one out of three respondents reported engaging in serious research misconduct (Wadman 2005). To prevent or counter misconduct, science has multiple lines of defense. The first line against misconduct is research training. Comprehensive scientific training covers technical skills and professional ethics encouraging honesty and integrity. The second line of defense includes the colleagues and laboratory partners who see day-to-day competence, successes, and failures. Colleagues are responsible for reporting concerns to authorities. Institutions are responsible for investigating reports of misconduct. Funders are another opportunity to intervene. Funding agency personnel regularly monitor funded studies in order to detect irregularities. While funders have the authority to stop funding or to press criminal charges for misconduct or fraud, businesses are less likely to intervene if the misconduct is in favor of the corporation's product. The next level of control, editorial and peer review, are designed to assess the quality of the research and to screen out questionable studies. An emerging issue is the recent explosion of online publishers allowing authors to bypass peer review. These vanity publishers often look and sound legitimate to the unsuspecting reader. A significant line of defense is journalists. To prevent spreading misinformation, journalists must act as investigators, double-checking sources, and filtering out misinformation. The last line of defense against bad science is the general public. Readers can prevent falling prey to disinformation or fraud by checking the accuracy of published research through multiple reputable sources. There are many opportunities to stop or prevent bad science. All of the systems must work together in order that science may benefit humanity.

PROFESSIONAL INTEGRITY OF RESEARCHERS

Experts agree that integrity starts with school, learning, and training (National Academy of Sciences, National Academy of Engineering, and Institute of Medicine 2009). However, school is hard work and humans like to find the most efficient way to achieve a desired outcome. Up to 64 percent of students report cheating in school (Simkin and McLeod 2010). Students cheat when they see education as a means to an end rather than an opportunity to exercise the brain and develop critical thinking. Consider the case of Elias A. K. Alsabti (chapter 1). After just three years of medical school, Alsabti realized that lying about his accomplishments was more efficient than studying. Anatomy and physiology, pathophysiology, biochemistry, pharmacology, and microbiology are not easy subjects. Alsabti was able to bypass hard work by falsely claiming credentials and stealing the work of other scientists. As a result, he enjoyed working at prestigious institutions. Alsabti's mentor, Al-Sayyab, modeled inappropriate behavior and his student took the behavior to the next level. There will always be some people who insist on taking shortcuts. Creating a culture of scientific integrity requires changes in the way teachers teach and mentors train. To promote academic integrity, education must focus on learning and reasoning as opposed to completing assignments (Chronicle of Higher Education 2018). To achieve this goal, teachers and professors are responsible for monitoring learning, detecting cheating in the classroom, and redirecting undesirable behavior. When the teacher overlooks cheating, other students will try to take shortcuts and cheating becomes endemic throughout the institution and to other institutions as students move on to college or graduate school.

While encouraging honest learning may promote integrity among many scientists in training, there is a small percentage of the population that believe they are above normal social rules. Psychologists identify the *Dark Triad* of personality disorders as a group of antisocial personality types focused on their own benefit and wants. The Dark Triad consists of narcissism, psychopathy, and Machiavellianism. One percent of the population suffers from narcissistic personality disorder (NPD) (Dhawan et al. 2010). NPD is characterized by a deep need for admiration combined with a lack of empathy for other people. Superficially, narcissists are charming and friendly. They crave attention and adoration and appear likeable because they want to keep their admirers paying deference to their many exaggerated accomplishments. When and if someone questions the narcissist, the daggers come out. The NPD can exhibit severe antisocial tendencies and lack remorse for their actions. Caught in a lie, the NPD will lash out with counterattack exhibiting very little empathy for the target of attack. Psychopaths exhibit similar traits as narcissists except they enjoy hurting other people. Psychopathic personalities are sadistic (see chapter 2, Josef Mengele). The Machiavellian personality is manipulative and deceitful. They will single-mindedly find ways to exploit others. The lack of direct supervision in research combined with high rewards is attractive to intelligent people with Dark Triad personality disorders. They are able to pursue their goal of admiration, attention, resources, money, power, and control in the academic world more easily than in other jobs. The personality traits and misconduct may eventually catch up to the perpetrator. In the meantime, a great deal of damage may be done to study participants, colleagues, institutions, and the general public who depend on scientists to act with integrity.

Some researchers start with the best of values and intentions and then gradually become corrupted by the business of science. In the *Chronicle of Higher Education*, professor of law at Harvard University Lawrence Lessig (2018) notes, "The thief knows he's a thief. But the good person doesn't." Georgetown University professors Sunita Sah and Adriane Fugh-Berman (2013) list and describe the many social processes that corrupt good people: confirmation bias, belief-in-self bias, entitlement bias, reciprocity bias, social-validation bias, and moral-license bias. Confirmation bias is the tendency to seek information that supports current views (see chapter 6, Confirmation Bias). Belief-in-self bias is the perception that one is not influenced by product marketing. Entitlement bias is the belief that one has worked hard to earn rewards and benefits and deserves nice things. Reciprocity bias is an obligatory exchange. If someone gives a gift, there is an expectation that the receiver owes the gift-giver. Social-validation bias is the idea that if peers accept gifts, the individual may also accept gifts. Likewise, if peers shun gifts, the individual should shun gifts. Moral-license bias is the idea that good deeds are stockpiled and many good deeds negate minor misbehaviors. With so many social norms supporting corruption, it is easy to see why and how even principled researchers are vulnerable to research misconduct.

Research and the interaction with human study participants requires the highest level of personal and professional integrity. To support responsible research, the UK Research Integrity Office (2009) published the *Code of Practice for Researchers*. General principles of ethical research practice are:

- *Excellence:* Researchers should strive to create work of the highest quality.

- *Honesty:* Researchers should report results with accuracy, acknowledge the contributions of others, avoid engaging in misconduct, and acknowledge limitations and mistakes.

- *Integrity:* Researchers must comply with legal, moral, and professional guidelines for practice, protect human study participants, and take steps to avoid or resolve conflict of interest.

- *Cooperation:* Within the constraint of study participant privacy, researchers should engage in open discussion and exchange of ideas.

- *Accountability:* Researchers should realize that they are ultimately responsible to the general public and must adhere to the requirements of professional practice and governing bodies.

- *Training and Skills:* Researchers are responsible for obtaining the necessary training required to carry out the proposed research.

- *Safety:* Researchers must ensure the rights and welfare of all study volunteers and avoid unreasonable risk or harm to study participants.

These principles encourage researchers to consider the wider implications of their work and to know and understand the power of scientific authority. Following these guidelines promotes public trust in scientists.

Scientists are responsible for accurately conveying new research findings to the public. To ensure that research is properly vetted by peers, scientists should wait until their work has passed through peer review before publicizing findings. If the study results have clinical implications, patients/study participants should be informed of the results before media outlets. In speaking to journalists, scientists should give a clear, accurate account of their work and avoid overgeneralizing or adding personal opinion. Scientists can prevent misinformation by helping journalists convey information accurately to the public.

PROTECTING WHISTLE-BLOWERS

Colleagues, students, and laboratory personnel are often the first people to notice questionable research practices. Seven out of 10 researchers report witnessing questionable scientific practices by colleagues (Fanelli 2009). However, very few are willing to risk their job or reputation to report misconduct. A whistle-blower is defined as someone who reveals information on illegal or unethical activities within a company or institution. In *Fortune* magazine, Patricia Sellers (2014) suggests that women are more likely to become whistle-blowers. Acting on the desire to nurture others regardless of personal cost, Sellers calls this the "motherhood gene," an innate drive to protect and defend those who are vulnerable. Sellers speculates this may be because women are more risk-aversive than men. Females identify the potential drawbacks of misconduct, whereas men see potential benefits. To compound gender differences, many business executives and scientists are males. Excluded from the corporate and science world, women are outsiders with an inside view to witnessing corruption, misconduct, and incompetence. Although women are more likely to report misconduct, they are also judged more harshly for reporting it. Female whistle-blowers are often dismissed or ridiculed and accused of being unreasonable, emotional, or too demanding.

Scholars at the University of Québec at Montreal identified four types of whistle-blowers: protective, skeptical, role-prescribed and self-interested (Smaili and Arroyo 2019). Protective whistle-blowers are interested in protecting the organization, society, or themselves. They have an idyllic view of science and that all scientists should practice with honesty and integrity. When they observe misconduct, they are often surprised and cautious in making accusations. Tyler Shultz (chapter 1, Elizabeth Holmes and Sunny Balwani), Walter DeNino (chapter 6, Eric Poehlman), and Bradford Perez (chapter 7, Anil Potti, Joseph Nevins, and Duke University officials) are examples of the protective whistle-blower. Protective whistle-blowers report concerns internally before going outside of the organization. Skeptical whistle-blowers are suspicious of the organization and do not believe that the regular channels of reporting will work to stop the misconduct. Skeptical whistle-blowers will report concerns to outsiders. Role-prescribed whistle-blowers are people who are outside of the organization and responsible for monitoring or uncovering irregularities. Role-prescribed whistle-blowers are motivated to report because it is part of their job. They could get in trouble for failing to report. Peter Buxton (chapter 2, U.S. Public Health Service and the Tuskegee Syphilis Study) is an example of the role-prescribed whistle-blower. Self-interested whistle-blowers are individuals who believe they can benefit from reporting misconduct. These whistle-blowers may sue the company for millions of dollars. Knowing and understanding the types of whistle-blowers is useful information in understanding motivations and reasons for reporting.

Dr. Nancy Olivieri is an example of a protective whistle-blower. In 1989, Olivieri was working at University of Toronto testing the drug deferiprone as a treatment for thalassemia. Thalassemia is a genetic disorder characterized by severe anemia. The pharmaceutical company Apotex partially funded the clinical trial. When study participants complained of adverse effects, Olivieri became concerned. She immediately notified the University of Toronto ethics board of the adverse events. She also intended to inform the study participants of the adverse events. However, Apotex intervened claiming that Olivieri had signed a nondisclosure agreement and that she would violate the legal agreement if she notified study participants. Olivieri did notify the study participants and Apotex responded with a concentrated effort to damage her reputation and discredit her. Olivieri remained firm in her conviction that participants should know the adverse effects of the experimental drug. In 2009, Olivieri was awarded American Association for the Advancement of Science (AAAS) Scientific Freedom and Responsibility Award "for her indefatigable determination that patient safety and research integrity come before institutional and commercial interests" (AAAS n.d.).

Perpetrators are attracted to systems that will accept improper behavior. They may groom the people around them to overlook misconduct. Dr. Kenneth B. Sloan is another well-known whistle-blower. Sloan's colleague, Nicholas S. Boder, professor at the University of Florida, invented a chemical delivery system (CDS) to transport medicine across the blood-brain barrier. The delivery system worked by attaching a special fat-soluble molecule to the desired medication. The compound was potentially very valuable because it could take chemicals past the blood-brain barrier into the brain. The product could potentially be used for AIDS, cancer, herpes, epilepsy, life-threatening infections, tranquilizers, fertility hormones, or chemicals required to image the brain for scans. Boder signed an exclusive license to market CDS through a new startup, Pharmatec. Pharmatec immediately signed agreements with Burroughs Welcome, DuPont, Pfizer, Nova Pharmaceutical, and Nedco Research. Of the $6 million in startup funds, Boder received $1 million for product development. While working as vice president and director of Pharmatec, Boder continued to hold his position as chairperson of the Department of Medicinal Chemistry at the University of Florida, College of Pharmacy. Pharmatec hired several faculty members from the medicinal chemistry department and gave company stocks to university faculty and the dean. Department colleagues and the dean served on Pharmatec's advisory board. One of the board members, Sloan noticed that the CDS molecule was structurally similar to a known toxin. Sloan suggested toxicology testing on primates before students or staff handled the chemical. The board members initially dismissed the suggestion. Sloan ended up resigning from the board and was later given a negative employee review (McGarity and Wagner 2008; Shamoo and Resnik 2009). The testing did eventually occur and Pharmatec went out of business. The case shows how easily potential whistle-blowers are corrupted by reciprocity bias.

Whistle-blowing is dangerous. When suspected or detected, perpetrators will often deny, claim ignorance, counterattack, threaten, belittle, blame others, or seek retribution. Whistle-blowing can result in bullying victimization, loss of funding support, termination of research contracts, and other forms of retaliation. With one's career or life work at stake, whistle-blowing takes a great deal of courage and tenacity. To protect and support would-be whistle-blowers, The Government Accountability Project offers these tips for whistle-blowers:

- Consider the big picture: Does the action meet the definition of misconduct? Is the allegation verifiable? Is the whistle-blower able to withstand attack? Are there things the whistle-blower has done that could be used against them?

- Make a plan and take action on your own time, not company time. Review company policy regarding the storage and distribution of documents. Secure any documents without attracting suspicion. Keep a detailed report of your own performance reviews.

- Consult with family members regarding potential financial or social implications. Consider all of the ways that the coworker or company could retaliate. Recognize that anything is possible.

- Consider working within the system and seek legal guidance as needed.
- Gently test coworkers to see how they respond to reporting. Build a supportive network outside of the office.
- Put the concern in writing and give evidence to support the concern. Do not exaggerate the accusation. Remain unemotional.
- Be patient. Give authorities sufficient time to investigate and accept that you may never know the outcome of the investigation.

In some institutions, failure to blow the whistle could be a violation of the institution's business code of conduct policy. Overlooking plagiarism or duplicate publishing so that a colleague can gain tenure or promotion is misappropriation of the institution's assets. Role-prescribed whistle-blowers do not have a choice in blowing the whistle. To protect whistle-blowers, the Office of Research Integrity outlines the rights and responsibilities of whistle-blowers as:

- Freedom to communicate reasonable concerns to authorities
- Timely investigation of the complaint
- Fair and impartial procedures for resolving complaints
- The ability to comment on the accuracy and completeness of the report documenting the whistle-blower's account
- Protection from retaliation
- Vindication of the complainant in cases where reports of misconduct are substantiated

Despite such rights, it is often difficult to go up against an individual or a system that benefit from misconduct. Furthermore, people who lie and cheat do not live by the same social rules and norms as others. If someone is willing to lie and cheat on the job, retaliation is not out of bounds. The federal government encourages whistle-blowers to report misconduct perpetrated in government grant-funded research through qui tam lawsuits. If the perpetrator is found guilty of defrauding the government, the whistle-blower is entitled to some of the funds recovered by the federal government.

One of the heroes in the fight against predatory publishing is librarian Jeffrey Beall, a role-prescribed whistle-blower. In 2008, Beall noticed an unusual number of requests asking him to serve on the editorial boards of what initially seemed to be scholarly journals. On closer inspection, Beall noticed that the messages contained terrible grammar. The poor grammar seemed highly unusual. These were supposed to be companies brokering professional publications. The journal names sounded legitimate. Beall quickly realized that some of the journals mimicked the names of well-known professional journals. For example, the American College of Obstetricians and Gynecologists publishes the journal,

Obstetrics & Gynecology. OMICS Group Inc. started the journal, *Gynecology & Obstetrics.* OMICS charges $5,000 for a one-year membership. One-year members can submit up to 18 articles to any of the OMICS journals. To warn academics against publishing in these venues Beall started a list of "potential, possible, or predatory scholarly open-access publishers." Beall's list quickly grew to hundreds of predatory open access journals. His list included explanations of how the journal met his criteria for predatory publishing. For example, in 2014, Scientific Research Publishing (SCIRP) published an article in their journal *Health* professing AIDS denialism. SCIRP currently charges $1,199 to publish in *Health.* Beall's list reported SCIRP as a possible predatory publisher because AIDS denialism is junk science that harms AIDS research, treatment, and prevention. (SCIRP later retracted the article.) As Beall's fight against predatory publishers gained attention, some of the groups tried to silence him. Predatory publishing brings in a lot of money. *Health* reports publishing 2,149 articles between 2009 and 2019. At $1,199 per article, that calculates to over $2.5 million and SCIRP lists over 200 open-access, online journals!

Many of the predatory publishers are based overseas. The immediate criticism was that Beall was biased against non-English-speaking publishers. As he continued his mission, he was subjected to legal threats and attacks. In 2013, OMICS threatened to sue Beall for $1 billion in damages. Beall's employer, University of Colorado refused to support him. In January 2017, Beall removed his list from the Internet. Copies of the list are archived on several websites. The closure of Beall's list is a failure for science and scientific publishing. Other groups are stepping up to champion the cause. Cabell's Scholarly Analytics recently started the Journal Blacklist to call out exploitive operations. The blogs, Flaky Academic Conferences and Flaky Academic Journals highlight e-mails inviting Professor David Kaye of Pennsylvania State University to submit papers. The invitations typically contain poor grammar and are aiming for a large number of submissions rather than quality submissions. Quackwatch is a network of volunteers managed by Dr. Stephen Barrett. The group monitor questionable health claims to advocate for responsible and accurate health information on the internet. Stop Predatory Journals is an anonymous group of scholars listing hijacked, predatory, and misleading journals. Retraction Watch monitors and records recent journal retractions as well as the stories behind the retraction. In 2016, the U.S. Federal Trade Commission, Bureau of Consumer Protection filed a civil complaint against OMICS. The FTC claimed that OMICS committed fraud by tricking researchers into paying fees for publication, listing individuals as editors who never agreed to edit the journals, and not disclosing fees in advance. OMICS responded that there was no fraud because the contributors knew that they were paying to publish and since OMICS was based in India, they were outside the jurisdiction of the FTC. In 2019, a federal judge ruled in favor of the FTC and imposed a $50.1 million fine on OMICS. Experts note that the main way to stop predatory publishing is to starve them out. As long as scientists pay to publish on these websites, the businesses will flourish. Shutting down predatory publishers will require concerted effort by academics, journalists, institutions, and the public.

INSTITUTIONAL CULTURE

While many institutions would prefer to look the other way when misconduct occurs, news of misconduct or scandal does impact institutional reputation and create the potential for lawsuit. For example, Ward Churchill (chapter 8) and James Tracy (chapter 8) both embarrassed their home institutions. University of Illinois at Chicago had to return $3.1 million in research grants awarded to Mani Pavuluri (chapter 5). With the assistance of bioethicist and lawyer, Alan Milstein, the Gelsinger family sued the University of Pennsylvania and settled for an undisclosed amount (chapter 6). Scandals influence college admissions, grant funding, and the ability to recruit strong scholars. Experts estimate that extensive media coverage of higher education scandal reduces the number of new applications by ten slots in the *U.S. News and World Report* rankings (Luca, Rooney, and Smith 2016). Decreases in applications mean less tuition revenue and more students with lower academic potential. While many institutions have policies against student misconduct, fewer have clear policies and procedures on faculty or administrator misconduct, and policies that do exist are easily overlooked if the researcher brings funding or prestige to the institution or has a strong network of peer support within the institution.

The current climate of decreased government funding for higher education pushes administrators to seek revenue elsewhere. Corporations, individuals, and other private sources are eager to use the knowledge, skills, and social authority of researchers. However, private funders often see the transaction as a business transaction. Research becomes a way to market a product or forward a political agenda rather than expand knowledge. Academic institutions must carefully consider the cost of corporate partnerships. Corporate partnerships tarnish public faith in science. Researchers at Brigham and Women's Hospital in Boston found that physicians were half as willing to prescribe drugs tested in industry-funded clinical trials compared to drugs studied in NIH-funded clinical trials (Kesselheim et al. 2012). Industry sponsorship negatively influenced the physicians' impressions of the quality of the study and the study outcomes. The loss of faith in science will eventually transfer to the institutions that depend heavily on corporate-sponsored research. To prevent corruption, institutions will have to develop stronger internal controls such as that at the University of Chicago where faculty recipients of summer research grants are not told who funded the grant until the end of the summer (Lessig 2018).

The first step in institutional responsibility is to create a culture of competence and integrity. The process starts by filtering out faculty applicants who do not have formal training in research. In an effort to cut costs, many institutions are trending toward teaching faculty, faculty who are trained in a particular field without formal research training. The advantage of teaching faculty is that they are less expensive and can help students make connections to practical content. Expecting someone without formal training in research to perform research is irresponsible. Ward Churchill (chapter 8) was hired because he brought publicity to the institution. He did not have the skills or interest in doing proper scholarship. When the lack of training in research comes up against the institutional requirements of faculty to perform research, individuals are tempted to take shortcuts and do not understand the implications of shortcuts. There needs to be a balance in the hiring process where both administration and experienced researchers have a voice in faculty hiring and rank. There also needs to be careful reflection and consideration of implicit biases. Too many highly qualified women and persons of color are overlooked because they do not fit the traditional image of a scientist.

To help institutions investigate allegations of misconduct, the UK Research Integrity Office (UKRIO) and the U.S. Office of Research Integrity provide detailed resources, sample institutional policy, and a flow chart on investigating and handling cases of misconduct. Under the UKRIO recommendations, each institution should have a named person responsible for receiving and responding to allegations of misconduct. The named person should be someone who will act with integrity and honesty, someone who is above institutional politics. The named person must review the nature of the allegation and immediately act to prevent harm to staff, study participants, or animals. If applicable, the named person must notify any regulatory or legal authority. If an investigation is warranted, a board of investigators is created. The investigators should review the study protocol and study materials, interview witnesses and the accused, and review study correspondence, data spreadsheets, and publications or conference presentations. If the investigators conclude a finding of misconduct, consequences are determined by the institution and the funding agency. Possible consequences include loss of funding, dismissal, journal retraction, fines, or criminal charges related to fraud. The key to avoiding the investigative process is to create an institutional culture of excellence, honesty, and integrity that discourages misconduct and takes appropriate action when and if misconduct occurs.

There is the need to expand and strengthen institutional responses. Currently, the only formal system of tracking misconduct is for scientists working on federal grants or through journal retractions. There is no formal system that tracks unscrupulous researchers outside of federal grants. This means that researchers who engage in misconduct outside of government grants are free to move to other organizations (see chapter 1, Elias Asabti).

PROFESSIONAL JOURNAL EDITORS

Publication in professional journals influences the care of thousands of patients and determines billions of dollars in medical treatment. The peer review system, if done correctly, allows colleagues to review, assess, and provide feedback on study results. The eventuality of peer review should encourage the author to present study methods and results honestly. However, peer reviews are limited in that reviewers can only assess what is in front of them. The scientist who engages in intentional misconduct may go out of the way to conceal misconduct. Pranks, such as the Sokal hoax, Sokal Squared, and the Star Wars midi-chlorian paper demonstrate weaknesses in the peer review process (see chapter 3). The system of professional research publishing—hoping the author is telling the truth—is naive. Based on their experiences with Boldt, the editors of *Anesthesia and Analgesia* revised their review process (see chapter 7). The updated practice requires authors to submit documentation that the study was approved by an ethics committee. All coauthors must sign a statement explaining how they contributed to the project, confirming that they saw the original study data, and naming potential or actual conflicts of interest. Clinical trials should be registered on a recognized clinical trials registry and data made available for review by other researchers. Editors should not be embarrassed or afraid to retract articles. To support editors, the International Committee of Medical Journal Editors (ICMJE) and Committee on Publication Ethics (COPE) provide guidelines suggesting best practices and recommendations on handling allegations of misconduct, plagiarism, manipulated images, redundant publication, or other misconduct. COPE guidelines include:

- Manuscript acceptance or rejection should be based on scope of the journal, importance and originality of the project, and clarity of the study.

- Studies that challenge current beliefs and studies with negative results should receive fair and unbiased consideration.

- Editorial decisions should not be influenced by advertisers.

- All original research studies should undergo full peer review.

- The manuscript and peer feedback should be handled confidentially.

- If problems are discovered in a published article, the editors must correct the information promptly and publicly.

If the editor believes a submission involves misconduct, the editor has an ethical obligation to act. The editor should not simply reject the manuscript and allow the submission to be passed on to another journal. If the author appears to have a genuine lack of understanding of scientific integrity, the editor has a responsibility to educate the author. If the misconduct is deeply concerning, the editor must decide whether to contact the author's employer, funder, or professional licensing board. Authors should be given the opportunity to respond to allegations of misconduct. Possible sanctions for misconduct include a letter of reprimand, publication of a notice of plagiarism, refusal to accept future submissions from the author, formal retraction of the publication, report to the author's employer, and report to the governing professional board.

As technology advances, there may be opportunities for editors to screen submissions. Students and scholars at Massachusetts Institute of Technology (MIT) originally created the software program SCIgen as a joke. The program randomly collects scientific jargon, patches phrases together, and creates figures to mimic a scientific paper. The papers are actually collections of meaningless gibberish. In 2010, Cyril Labbé used SCIgen to generate 102 papers. Labbé also created a fictitious author in Google Scholar, Ike Antkare. Antkare scored a Google Scholar citation index of 94, ranking him as the 21st most highly cited scientist in the world (Van Noorden 2014). Labbé then turned his attention to identifying computer-generated papers published between 2008 and 2013. As a result of Labbé's review, the Institute of Electrical and Electronics Engineers (IEEE) and Springer retracted more than 120 papers from their databases. Labbé reports that SCIgen papers are easy to detect because they use characteristic vocabulary. Labbé's software can be used to detect nonsense papers in much the same way that plagiarism detection software identifies plagiarism. In the future, this type of software program may be used to weed out nonsense or fabricated research.

GOVERNMENT AGENCIES

As a primary funder of health and medical research, the federal government oversees many research studies. The Office of Research Integrity (ORI) acts on behalf of the Secretary of Health and Human Services to oversee research funded by the National Institutes of Health, Centers for Disease Control and Prevention, Substance Abuse Mental Health Services Administration, and other Public Health Service agencies, excluding the Food and Drug Administration. ORI develops policies related to the detection and investigation of allegations of misconduct, recommends administrative action, supports institutions responding to allegations, and conducts policy analyses. The overall purpose of ORI activities is to prevent misconduct and promote scientific integrity in order to maintain public trust in science. The ORI website tracks and publishes case summaries of research misconduct findings.

If research misconduct facilitates fraud against state or federal government, the government agency can require a Corporate Integrity Agreement. A Corporate Integrity Agreement lists specific obligations required to prevent a company from being banned from federal health care programs, such as Medicare and Medicaid services. In the *New England Journal of Medicine*, lawyer Kevin Outterson (2012) questions the power of Corporate Integrity Agreements. Outterson notes that of the top 10 pharmaceutical companies, 8 were under Corporate Integrity Agreements with the federal government. Under the multimillion-dollar Paxil settlement, GlaxoSmithKline (GSK) was required to agree to a five-year Corporate Integrity Agreement with the Department of Health and Human Services, Office of Inspector General (see chapter 3). The goal of the agreement was to ensure individual accountability of the GSK board and executives. The main components of the agreement were changes in the way that the GSK sales force is compensated, allowing the company to recoup annual bonuses from current and former GSK executives and other GSK employees who engage in significant misconduct, and greater transparency in research practices and publications. The settlement stopped short of bringing criminal charges against named individuals. Outterson points out that pharmaceutical companies are earning billions of dollars in drug sales. Fines may simply become part of the cost of business.

JOURNALISTS

Through honest and investigative reporting, journalists can fill an incredible and very necessary role in society. For example, Allen Hornblum documented Kligman's dermatological studies in his book, *Acres of Skin: Human Experiments at Holmesburg Prison* (see chapter 5). Rebecca Skloot reported the life, history, and injustices surrounding the HeLa cell line in *The Immortal Life of Henrietta Lacks* (chapter 6). Alicia Mundy described Wyeth's attempts to cover up the adverse effects of a diet drug in *Dispensing with the Truth: The Victims, the Drug Companies, and the Dramatic Story behind the Battle over Fen-Phen* (chapter 7). The first step to good investigative journalism is maintaining a sense of healthy skepticism and not falling for the charismatic demo doll who offers a fascinating human-interest story or presents a research study that seems too good to be true. To prevent disseminating misinformation, journalists should check the credentials of their source, consider whether the claims or promises are credible, verify facts with independent, reliable sources, and understand the limitations of science and scientific studies. Best journalistic practices include:

- Consider how the information affects the reader.
- Question whether a story is accurate as well as newsworthy.
- Investigate the entire story through reputable sources. Avoid getting information from commercial sources.
- Consult with people who have studied the topic or published in the field. Avoid self-professed experts.
- Present the story using accurate and impartial facts.

- Go beyond the headlines to include subtle, nuanced information. Avoid oversimplifying.

- When reporting on a story involving health issues, such as heart disease, suicide, domestic violence, or substance abuse, include practical advice, hotlines, and resources.

- Avoid presenting new technology, treatment, or medicine as a magic solution.

- Avoid blaming the victim.

Red flags for questionable sources include lack of focus of the resource, extremely broad scope of topics, and poor grammar. Journalists are in a great position to stop misinformation.

PUBLIC MEDIA AWARENESS

Information is power. False information may be used to market a product, create confusion, or divide communities. Marketing, fake news, rumors, hoaxes, and disinformation play on people's emotions in order to manipulate behavior. *The Disinformation Playbook* by the Union of Concerned Scientists describes five strategies used by companies to influence consumer behavior:

- Presenting content that appears to be based on legitimate research but is based on counterfeit science

- Harassing and intimidating scientists who threaten the corporation's bottom line

- Creating doubt about research that finds a product may be harmful to consumers

- Collaborating with legitimate professional groups and scientists to create a screen of legitimacy

- Manipulating government organizations to create policies that directly or indirectly support corporate interests

Misinformation is harmful because it destroys community cohesion. The most obvious sign of misinformation is poorly written text, stock photos, and multiple spelling or grammar mistakes. Imposters tend to have a large volume of postings with very little personal information. It is difficult to trace the author's background.

As social media outlets begin to recognize the impact of false information, companies are attempting to control divisive and destructive messages. The best way to stop attacks, urban myths, and other nonsense from spreading is for members of the public to recognize the misinformation and to stop forwarding it. Readers are encouraged to fact check, read beyond the initial reference to look at other reputable sources, read with skepticism, and not to fall for the illusion of explanatory depth or confirmation biases. Experts recommend the following steps to improve media literacy:

- Consider the source. Check out primary sources. Check the author, check the date, and check links.

- Understand the methods of marketers, predatory publishers, and others engaged in pushing misinformation.

- Expand your knowledge of a topic. Do not disregard information just because it does not fit with current beliefs. Read articles with information that you do not agree with.

- Be skeptical of information that seems too good to be true. News is not a popularity contest. Likes or shares do not mean the story is accurate.

- Call out yellow journalism. Immediately report inaccurate stories to the journalist or news site.

- Realize that scientists do not always agree.

- Understand the difference between correlation and cause.

The Finnish people are a good model for media awareness. In 2014, the Finnish government launched an initiative teaching students, citizens, journalists, and policy makers how to recognize fake news. Students are encouraged to investigate information before they pass it on to others, to check information against other credible sources and avoid collecting information from alternative news sites, such as Facebook, Twitter, Google, YouTube, or Instagram. Finland also worked on developing a strong sense of who they are as a country. As a result, Finland ranks highest in recognizing fake news stories, refusing to perpetuate misinformation, and not being a soft target for internet trolls, disinformation, or bots. Journalist Jessikka Aro is credited with Finland's high media literacy. Aro educates people on how to identify false rumors, disinformation, and destructive posts. Through her work, Aro has experienced threats, assaults to her reputation, and was overlooked for awards. Society must find ways to protect and honor journalists who are willing to explore and report on the darker sides of humanity.

COMMUNITY PARTNERSHIPS

Community-engaged scholarship is collaboration between researchers in academic institutions and people in the local or regional community. Collaborative partners share information and resources in order to address a particular health or social issue of concern. The scientist works with key community members to identify concerns within the community, design a study, collect data, and regularly report back to community partners. Community-engaged research is different from traditional research in that the community members have a strong say in which problems are studied, how data will be collected, and how results will be used. The researcher is not elevated to a position of authority. The community and study participants are just as much authorities on the topic as the scientist and in most cases, the scientist learns from the community.

One example of community-engaged research is the case of the Flint water crisis. In 2003, a group of homeowners in Washington, D.C., called Virginia Tech professor Marc Edwards to investigate their drinking water. The environmental engineer found extraordinarily high levels of lead. The District of Columbia Water and Sewer Authority and the Environmental Protection Agency refuted Edwards's findings and pulled his research funding. In 2004, the *Washington Post* ran a front-page report on lead contamination in the D.C. water supply. Edwards testified before Congress on the cause and possible solutions to the problem. He is credited with going up against a bureaucratic system to advocate for public health and safety. In 2015, LeAnn Walters of Flint, Michigan asked Edwards to come to her home town and test her family's drinking water. Flint officials had switched the municipal water supply from Detroit to the less expensive Flint River supply. The water coming out of Walters's tap ranged from light to dark yellow. The family experienced abdominal pain, rashes, and hair loss. The city tested Walters's water and advised the family not to drink it due to high lead levels. As other residents complained, city officials insisted that the lead contamination was isolated to the Walters residence even though the Walters household had plastic pipes. Edwards visited Flint and collected water samples. He discovered lead levels up to 800 times the legal limit of 15 parts per billion (McQuaid 2016). Officials initially claimed that residents were contaminating their own water for attention. The Michigan Department of Environmental Quality denied there were problems with lead contamination and attempted to discredit Edwards. When Michigan State University professor and pediatrician Dr. Mona Hanna-Attisha published data showing that children's blood lead levels had almost doubled in the area, officials could no longer deny the problem. Michigan State budgeted $240 million for lead remediation and public health programs. Drinking water advisories were implemented to warn residents to use water filters. The lead levels have since decreased. The long-term effects of lead poisoning on the children of Flint remains to be seen.

Community-engaged scholarship is a unique form of research. Community-engaged scholars work outside of the laboratory or library. They must meet with and speak to numerous stakeholders in order to gain social and financial support. Edwards used his own money to support the initial research in Flint. When community-engaged scholars apply for tenure and promotion, their unique scholarship is often not recognized by reviewers on the board on rank and tenure. To differentiate community-based scholarship from community service, the

Community-Campus Partnerships for Health developed indicators of effective community-based scholarship (Jordan 2007):

- Disciplined preparation by the scholar in the area of interest
- A clear goal or goals for academic and community improvement
- Significant impact in the community, scholarly, and professional field
- Dissemination of results to communities as well as professional and popular media
- Evidence of leadership and professional integrity
- Synthesis of activities into research, teaching, and service

Community partnerships empower the community while helping the scientist to explore an issue through the experiences of those directly involved with the problem. Community-engaged research reduces the potential for scientific misconduct because the scientist has regular oversight and is responsible for reporting results to an engaged and interested community. Bringing science into the community helps both the scientist and society.

Unregulated pursuit of knowledge, yearning for recognition, and competition for funding create a system where some people will try to take shortcuts. Mentors, colleagues, institutions, journal editors, journalists, grant funders, and the public can create and support systems to encourage and promote scientific integrity. Through a collaborative, holistic, and honest approach, science can help humanity to advance.

FURTHER READING

AAAS (American Association for the Advancement of Science). n.d. "2009 Award for Scientific Freedom and Responsibility Recipient." Accessed August 21, 2019. https://www.aaas.org/awards/scientific-freedom-and -responsibility/2009

Alford, C. Fred. 2001. *Whistleblowers: Broken lives and Organizational Power.* Ithaca, NY: Cornell University Press.

Chronicle of Higher Education. 2018. "Building Academic Integrity." Accessed August 28, 2019. http://images.results.chronicle.com/Web/TheChronicle ofHigherEducation/%7Bf2096f09-89cf-400c-aca3-07dd6c6a81b5%7D _Academic_Integrity_CaseStudy_v4.pdf

Dhawan, Nikhil, Mark E. Kunik, John Oldham, and John Coverdale. 2010. "Prevalence and Treatment of Narcissistic Personality Disorder in the Community: A Systematic Review." *Comprehensive Psychiatry* 51 (4): 333–39.

Fanelli, Daniele. 2009. "How Many Scientists Fabricate and Falsify Research? A Systematic Review and Meta-Analysis of Survey Data." *PLoS ONE* 4 (5): 1–11.

Government Accountability Project. *Whistleblowing Survival Tips.* Accessed April 27, 2019. https://www.whistleblower.org/resources/#survival-tips

Jordan, Cathy. 2007. "Community-Engaged Scholarship Review, Promotion & Tenure Package." Peer Review Workgroup, Community-Engaged Scholarship for Health Collaborative, Community-Campus Partnerships for Health. Accessed April 27, 2019. https://www.ccphealth.org/wp-content /uploads/2017/10/CES_RPT_Package.pdf

Kesselheim, Aaron S., Christopher T. Robertson, Jessica A. Myers, Susannah L. Rose, Victoria Gillet, Kathryn M. Ross, Robert J. Glynn, Steven Joffe, and Jerry Avorn. 2012. "A Randomized Study of How Physicians Interpret Research Funding Disclosures." *New England Journal of Medicine* 367 (12): 1119–27.

Lessig, Lawrence. 2018. "How Academic Corruption Works." *Chronicle of Higher Education*, October 12. Accessed December 16, 2019. https:// search-ebscohost-com.ezproxy.sju.edu/login.aspx?direct=true&db=aph &AN=133020311&site=eds-live

Luca, Michael, Patrick Rooney, and Jonathan Smith. 2016. "The Impact of Campus Scandals on College Applications." *Working Papers—Harvard Business School Division of Research*, July, 183–84.

McGarity, Thomas O., and Wendy Elizabeth Wagner. 2008. *Bending Science: How Special Interests Corrupt Public Health Research.* Cambridge, MA: Harvard University Press.

McPhee, John. 2009. "Checkpoints." *New Yorker* 85 (1): 56–63.

McQuaid, John. 2016. "Without These Whistleblowers, We May Never Have Known the Full Extent of the Flint Water Crisis; A Concerned Mother and a Renowned Scientist Spearheaded the Investigation That Exposed the Dangers Lurking in the Water Supply of the Michigan City." *Smithsonian*, December 1. Accessed April 28, 2019. https://www.smith sonianmag.com/innovation/whistleblowers-marc-edwards-and-leeanne -walters-winner-smithsonians-social-progress-ingenuity-award -180961125/

National Academy of Sciences, National Academy of Engineering, and Institute of Medicine. 2009. *On Being a Scientist: A Guide to Responsible Conduct in Research.* 3rd ed. Washington, D.C.: The National Academies Press. https://doi.org/10.17226/12192

Office of Research Integrity. n.d. "Whistleblower's Bill of Rights." Accessed April 18, 2018. https://ori.hhs.gov/Whistleblower-Rights

Outterson, Kevin. 2012. "Punishing Health Care Fraud—Is the GSK Settlement Sufficient?" *New England Journal of Medicine* 367 (12): 1082–85.

Sah, Sunita, and Adriane Fugh-Berman. 2013. "Physicians under the Influence: Social Psychology and Industry Marketing Strategies." *Journal of Law, Medicine and Ethics: A Journal of the American Society of Law, Medicine and Ethics* 41 (3): 665–72.

Sellers, Patricia. 2014. "Are Women More Likely than Men to Be Whistleblowers?" *Fortune.Com*, October 1. Accessed November 21, 2019. http://fortune.com/2014/09/30/women-whistleblowers/

Shamoo, Adil E., and David B. Resnik. 2009. *Responsible Conduct of Research.* New York: Oxford University Press.

Simkin, Mark, and Alexander McLeod. 2010. "Why Do College Students Cheat?" *Journal of Business Ethics* 94 (3): 441–53.

Smaili, Nadia, and Paulina Arroyo. 2019. "Categorization of Whistleblowers Using the Whistleblowing Triangle." *Journal of Business Ethics* 157 (1): 95–117.

Smith, Richard. 2006. "Research Misconduct: The Poisoning of the Well." *Journal of the Royal Society of Medicine* 99 (5): 232–237.

Sprague, Robert L. 1993. "Whistleblowing: A Very Unpleasant Avocation." *Ethics & Behavior* 3 (1): 103–133.

Tavare, Aniket, and Fiona Godlee. 2012. "Tackling Research Misconduct." *British Medical Journal* 345 (7870): 9.

UK Research Integrity Office. 2009. "Code of Practice for Research: Promoting Good Practice and Preventing Misconduct." Accessed January 24, 2018. https://ukrio.org/wp-content/uploads/UKRIO-Code-of-Practice-for-Research.pdf

Union of Concerned Scientists Center for Science and Democracy. "The Disinformation Playbook: How Business Interests Deceive, Misinform, and Buy Influence at the Expense of Public Health and Safety." Accessed April 27, 2019. https://www.ucsusa.org/our-work/center-science-and-democracy/disinformation-playbook

Van Noorden, Richard. 2014. "Publishers Withdraw More than 120 Gibberish Papers." *Nature*, February 25. Accessed January 24, 2019. https://www.nature.com/news/publishers-withdraw-more-than-120-gibberish-papers-1.14763

Wadman, Meredith. 2005. "One in Three Scientists Confesses to Having Sinned." *Nature* 435 (7043): 718–719.

Ward, Philip. 2012. "Research Fraud Requires Urgent Action." *Applied Clinical Trials* 21 (2): 12.

Guide to Evaluating Health and Psychology Studies

The purpose of research in medicine and psychology is to improve how doctors, psychiatrists, and other health professionals diagnose, treat, and care for people who are ill or to discover the best ways to prevent illness and injury. The ability to read and evaluate research articles empowers the reader to determine whether the reported study should influence community or clinical health practices. Knowledge of the strengths and limitations of research strengthens consumer health by deconstructing misleading marketing. The most efficient way to critique research is to break the research down into various parts and assess each part individually and then as a whole. The questions below suggest points to consider in assessing a research article.

AUTHORS AND SOURCE

1. Who wrote the article? Can the author's credentials be confirmed by an independent source?

2. Where does the author work? Will the researcher or the researcher's employer benefit financially from the study results?

3. Who financed the study? Could the funder directly or indirectly influence study activities or data analysis and reporting?

4. Where was the article published? Is this source a reputable publisher, a commercial website, or popular media?

5. Did the author pay for publication? If so, does the cost of publication justify the amount paid? Does the amount seem high in comparison to publication fees?

6. Was the research manuscript reviewed by independent peers?

RESEARCH PROBLEM

1. What is the health problem being investigated?
2. How many people are impacted by this issue? What are the health and social consequences?
3. How will society benefit from the proposed research?
4. Does the literature review present sufficient evidence supporting the need for this study?
5. What is the primary research question?
6. What are the major research hypotheses?
7. How did the researcher operationalize their variables?
8. What are the ethics of the proposed research? How did the researchers protect human participants?

RESEARCH DESIGN AND METHODS

1. Who is the study population?
2. Is the study sample generalizable?
3. How did the researchers recruit or gather the study sample?
4. What biases exist in sample selection?
5. What is the research design of the study?
6. What research instruments did the researchers use?
7. Are the research instruments valid and reliable?
8. What study methods did the researchers follow?
9. How else could the researchers have collected data? What are alternative ways to study this topic?

RESULTS AND DISCUSSION

1. How are data analyzed?
2. How are data presented?
3. Are study results written a way that the reader can understand?
4. Do study results support the major conclusions of the study?
5. What are the implications of the research findings for practice?
6. What are the implications of the research findings for future research?
7. What are the major limitations of the study?

Directory of Resources

BOOKS

Berezow, Alex. 2017. *Little Black Book of Junk Science*. New York: American Council on Science and Health. Accessed November 22, 2019. https://www.acsh.org/sites/default/files/Little%20Black%20Book%20of%20Junk%20Science.pdf

Borel, Brooke. 2016. *The Chicago Guide to Fact-Checking*. Chicago Guides to Writing, Editing, and Publishing. Chicago: University of Chicago Press.

Broad, William, and Nicholas Wade. 1982. *Betrayers of the Truth: Fraud & Deceit in the Halls of Science*. New York: Simon & Schuster.

Goodstein, David L. 2010. *On Fact and Fraud: Cautionary Tales from the Front Lines of Science*. Princeton, NJ: Princeton University Press.

Gorman, Sara E., and Jack M. Gorman. 2017. *Denying to the Grave: Why We Ignore the Facts That Will Save Us*. New York: Oxford University Press.

Hornblum, Allen M. 1998. *Acres of Skin: Human Experiments at Holmesburg Prison: A Story of Abuse and Exploitation in the Name of Medical Science*. New York: Routledge.

Jones, J. H. 1981. *Bad Blood: The Tuskegee Syphilis Experiment*. New York: Free Press; London: Collier Macmillan Publishers.

Judson, Horace Freeland. 2004. *The Great Betrayal: Fraud in Science*. Orlando: Harcourt.

Park, Robert. 2000. *Voodoo Science: The Road from Foolishness to Fraud*. New York: Oxford University Press.

Skloot, Rebecca. 2010. *The Immortal Life of Henrietta Lacks*. New York: Crown Publishers.

ONLINE ARTICLES

Atomic Heritage Foundation. 2017. "Human Radiation Experiments." July 11. Accessed November 22, 2019. https://www.atomicheritage.org/history /human-radiation-experiments

European Commission. n.d. "Ethics." Accessed November 22, 2019. https://ec .europa.eu/programmes/horizon2020/en/h2020-section/ethics

National Institutes of Health. 2010. "Research Integrity." Accessed November 22, 2019. https://grants.nih.gov/grants/research_integrity/research_misconduct .htm

ORGANIZATIONS

American Association for the Advancement of Science (AAAS) (https://www.aaas.org/)

The mission of the AAAS is to facilitate international communication and cooperation between scientists, engineers, and the public, promote scientific integrity, give voice to science with respect to social issues, promote responsible use of science in public policy, and promote education in science and technology. AAAS encourages STEM education by providing resources and information to support students, teachers, and policy makers.

American Press Institute (API) (https://www.americanpressinstitute.org/)

Founded in 1946, the API's mission is to support news agencies in the First Amendment rights to free speech. The basic premise of API is that society needs accurate information in order to debate and solve problems. API supports publishers and journalists in engaging audiences, creating revenue to enable free press, promoting accountable journalism, and sharing business strategies and best practices.

American Psychological Association (APA) (http://www.apa.org/research/responsible/)

The APA is the leading organization of student and practicing psychology professionals. The APA website provides information on psychological science news and events and responsible conduct in psychological research.

Cabell's Scholarly Analytics (http://www.cabells.org/)

Cabell's is a searchable database of over 11,000 professional journals. Cabell's offers a Whitelist of academic journals describing journal metrics and impact, acceptance rates, and publishing activity of reputable scholarly journals as well as a blacklist of journals engaging in predatory publishing. Cabell's was designed to help academic boards determine the quality of publication in determining tenure and promotion decisions.

Committee on Publication Ethics (COPE) (https://publicationethics.org/)

COPE provides best practice guidelines to support editors and publishers in identifying and following ethical publishing practices. The website features flowcharts and core practices to guide editors in dealing with cases of peer review manipulation, image doctoring, questionable authorship, or other suspected scientific misconduct.

Council for International Organizations of Medical Sciences (CIOMS) (https://cioms.ch/)

The World Health Organization (WHO) and The United Nations Educational, Scientific and Cultural Organization (UNESCO) established CIOMS to advance public health. CIOMS provides guidance to the international biomedical scientific community on ethics of health research, medical product development, and safety.

Council of Science Editors (CSE) (https://www.councilscienceeditors.org/)

CSE is an international organization for scientific publishing professionals educating, networking, and discussing current and emerging issues in the communication of scientific information.

The Department of Bioethics of the National Institutes of Health (https://www.bioethics.nih.gov/home/index.shtml)

The Department of Bioethics of the National Institutes of Health is a leading center for training, research, and service related to bioethical issues. The department aims to build a supportive network of scholars. One daily tradition of the department is to gather for mid-afternoon tea and snacks and discussion of current bioethical issues.

FACTCHECK.ORG (https://www.factcheck.org/)

FactCheck.org is a project of The Annenberg Public Policy Center of the University of Pennsylvania designed to monitor news related to public policy and assess current news stories for factual accuracy.

Flaky Academic Conferences (http://flakyc.blogspot.com/)

Flaky Academic Conferences is an online repository of e-mails received by Professor David Kaye of Pennsylvania State University inviting his submission to questionable conferences. The blog and e-mails highlight the proliferation of deceptive practices and techniques used by scammers.

Government Accountability Project (https://www.whistleblower.org/)

The Government Accountability Project promotes corporate and government accountability by advocating for and supporting whistle-blowers. The resource has many helpful tips and proactive suggestions for those considering reporting scientific misconduct.

International Center for Academic Integrity (ICAI) (https://academicintegrity.org/)

The mission of ICAI is to combat cheating, plagiarism, and academic dishonesty in higher education by supporting and sharing research related to academic honesty standards and practices. The website offers a variety of resources including the booklet, "Fundamental Values of Academic Integrity."

National Association of Media Literacy Education (NAMLE) (https://namle.net/)

NAMLE aims to empower individuals by building critical thinking skills related to mass media, popular culture, and digital technologies.

National Coalition Against Censorship (NCAC) (https://ncac.org/)

The mission of the NCAC is to "promote freedom of thought, inquiry and expression and oppose censorship in all its forms." NCAC provides resources for students, teachers, parents, school officials, artists, curators, librarians, and activists to promote free expression and to challenge censorship.

Office of the Associate Director for Science (OADS) (https://www.cdc.gov/od/science/index.htm)

OADS advocates for the use of science to address important public health problems and promotes quality and integrity among Centers for Disease Control and Prevention/ Agency for Toxic Substances and Disease Registry scientists.

Office of Human Research Protections (OHRP) (https://www.hhs.gov/ohrp/)

OHRP provides clarification, guidance, and regulatory oversight on the protection and welfare of human study participants in research supported by the U.S. Department of Health and Human Services.

Office of Research Integrity (ORI) (https://ori.hhs.gov/)

The ORI oversees Public Health Service research on behalf of the U.S. Secretary of Health and Human Services. The ORI reviews, monitors, and investigates reports of research misconduct by scientists and institutions awarded research grants by the DHHS. The website lists cases of misconduct, summaries of the case, outcomes, and other materials dating back to 2005.

Quackwatch (http://www.quackwatch.org/)

Quackwatch is a network of volunteers with the mission of investigating questionable health claims, advising victims of health-related frauds or misconduct, reporting illegal marketing, and advocating for quality health information on the internet. The website is managed by Dr. Stephen Barrett with a group of dedicated volunteers. The site presents questionable therapies and possible scams.

Retractionwatch.com (http://retractionwatch.com/)

Retraction Watch is a blog of the Center for Scientific Integrity. The site provides news on recent scientific journal retractions, the stories behind the retractions, and information such as how to tell if an image has been manipulated. Retraction watch provides a free searchable database of retracted journal articles.

Scholars At Risk Network (https://www.scholarsatrisk.org/)

Scholars at Risk is an international network of individuals and institutions headquartered at New York University. The organization supports scholarship by protecting the freedom of scholars to think, question, and discuss controversial topics. Each year, Scholars at Risk supports approximately 300 scholars who have experienced threats, imprisonment, or retaliation for speaking out on political and social problems.

Snopes.com (https://www.snopes.com/)

Snopes was started in 1994 as a source for journalists and readers to fact check urban legends, hoaxes, and folklore. Snopes staff investigate reports, check sources, and document findings to allow readers to determine whether the story is trustworthy. The website contains timeless myths and tales as well as stories in the current news.

Stop Predatory Journals (https://predatoryjournals.com/about/)

Stop Predatory Journals is a group of scholars with the goal of promoting information literacy. The website lists hijacked journals, predatory journals, and misleading or fake metrics that indicate a publishing website may not be legitimate. The authors of the website prefer to remain anonymous to avoid harassment and threats by predatory publishers.

Union of Concerned Scientists (https://www.ucsusa.org/)

The Union of Concerned Scientists is a group of scientists, analysts, policy, and communication experts with the goal of using research-based decision making to create a healthier planet and safer world. The site features current news, blogs, and other resources reporting environmental threats and related environmental policies.

#WOMENALSOKNOWSTUFF (https://womenalsoknowstuff.com/) and #WOMENALSOKNOWHISTORY (https://womenalsoknowhistory.com/)

#WOMENALSOKNOWSTUFF and #WOMENALSOKNOWHISTORY are two different databases of scholars who identify as women. The purpose of the websites is to provide academics, journalists, researchers, conference planners, and editors with a list of potential scholars in order that female scholars are appropriately represented as experts in the discipline and popular media.

Glossary

Abductive reasoning: a form of logic that creates the most plausible explanation for a phenomenon based on available evidence.

Abstract: a written summary of a research article.

Academic: related to education or scholarship.

Adverse event: an undesirable experience by one or more study participants as a result of the study.

Bench marking: a strategy of comparing a product, process, or workflow to best practices in a similar but unrelated field.

Conditions of causality: criteria defined by scientists to support the idea that one factor (the causal factor) generates or determines a second factor (the outcome variable).

Confirmation bias: the tendency to seek, interpret, or record results that support the scientist's existing beliefs or theory.

Contract publishing: an emerging term that sometimes refers to vanity publishing or ghostwriting.

Contract research organization (CRO): an independent contractor sponsored by a pharmaceutical or biotechnology company to design, select, manage, evaluate, and prepare study documents for product approval by the Food and Drug Administration.

Data: facts, statistics, or other information collected for reference or analysis.

Data analysis: the process of reviewing, cleaning, and transforming information in order to draw conclusions or discover new information.

Data conversion: the process of changing data from one format to another format. Data conversion typically refers to exporting data from one software program to another where the data may be more easily handled.

Datum: singular form of data.

Declaration of Helsinki: ethical principles for human participant research established by the World Medical Association.

Deductive reasoning: a form of logic that flows from a general idea to a specific conclusion.

Duplicate publishing: publishing the same intellectual material multiple times typically for the purpose of increasing the number of publications or distorting citation impact (*see also* redundant publishing and self-plagiarism).

Empirical: based on direct observation or experience.

Empiricism: the idea that all knowledge derives from the senses of hearing, seeing, smelling, tasting, touching, and experiencing.

Ethics dumping: the exploitation of populations in low-income countries by researchers from middle-income countries in order to avoid best practices in human participant protections.

Fabrication: making up study results and presenting the results as actual research findings.

Falsification: manipulating research instruments, procedures, or study results so that the research findings no longer reflect the final actual results.

Fraud: the intentional deception of others for personal or financial gain of the perpetrator

Humanism: a way of thinking about the world and other people that assumes humans are innately good and world problems may be alleviated through science.

Inductive reasoning: a form of logic that observes and examines the experiences, attitudes, behavior, or knowledge of a sample of individuals in order to generalize ideas to a larger group of people.

Junk science: a nonspecific term that refers to useless misinformation related to pseudoscience or fraud.

Literature review: a summary of the published information on a particular topic.

Longitudinal study: examines the same group of research participants over time to detect trends in the variable of interest.

Manels: scientific panels favoring male speakers while dismissing female scholars.

Mega journal: a large, peer-reviewed open access journal with lower selectivity than traditional print journals.

Meta-analysis: a statistical analysis of the pooled results of separate but similar studies in order to estimate effect size.

Nuremberg Code: a set of ethical principles designed to protect human study participants in biomedical research.

Open access publishing: online, free articles published by conventional publishers.

Pathological science: unintentional self-delusion by scientists.

Plagiarism: the act of intentionally taking credit for the words, ideas, or work of another person; from the Latin word *plagiarius* meaning "literary thief."

Population: a large collection of individuals or elements that is the subject of scientific inquiry.

Predatory publishing: an exploitive or deceptive publishing where article processing charges greatly exceed the actual cost of managing the operation. Predatory publishers tend to offer low-quality services to upload articles to a website.

Primary investigator: lead researcher on a grant-funded project.

Protocol: a document that clearly describes the background, purpose, design, methods, and data analysis of a study and how the results will be used.

Pseudoscience: part science, part nonsense.

Qualitative: related to the nature or quality of an experience, appearance, or situation.

Quantitative: related to numbers or measurement.

Qui tam lawsuit: a lawsuit that rewards whistle-blowers for reporting fraud against the federal government. Qui tam is taken from the Latin phrase "qui tam pro domino rege quam pro se ipso in hac parte sequitur," which means "he who brings an action for the king as well as himself."

Redundant publishing: publishing substantial sections of a previously published work more than once (*see also* duplicate publishing and self-plagiarism).

Research misconduct: intentional fabrication, falsification, or plagiarism that occurs during the scientific process.

Retraction: a withdrawal from the scientific literature.

Rogeting: a form of plagiarism where the plagiarist replaces one or two words or phrases of original text with synonyms from *Roget's Thesaurus* so that plagiarism detection software does not match the revised text with the original source.

Self-plagiarism: the reuse of one's own previous work without citing the original publication.

Self-publishing: the publication of an article, book, or other material at one's own financial expense.

Skew: distorted from the true value, statistically asymmetrical or giving an inaccurate representation.

Statement of the problem: part of the literature review that describes why a particular issue is important to individuals, communities, or society and worth studying.

Statistical significance: a result that is not likely to be due to random chance.

Study participant: individuals who volunteer and consent to be part of a research study.

Study sample: a subset of a population used to represent the entire population.

Study subject: an outdated term referring to a study participant.

Toll-access: a journal where the reader must pay to access the journal either as hard copy or electronically or through a library.

Vanity publishing: when authors pay a company to publish their book, article, or other written work.

Variable: a characteristic or factor that changes.

Whistle-blower: a person who exposes illicit activity within an organization.

Index

About the Author

Sally Kuykendall, PhD, is professor of health services at Saint Joseph's University, a community-based researcher, and a former nurse. She is author of *Bullying*, in Greenwood's Health and Medical Issues Today series, and editor of the *Encyclopedia of Public Health: Principles, People, and Programs*. She serves on the editorial advisory board of ABC-CLIO's Health and Wellness Issues: Understanding Science, Society, and Yourself database. Sally lives outside of Philadelphia, Pennsylvania with her husband and grandpuppies.